Self-Study Exercises in Radiography

Self-Study Exercises in Radiography

William L. Leonard, MA, RT, (R)
Associate Professor of Allied Health
and
Radiography Program Director
Bergen Community College
Paramus, New Jersey

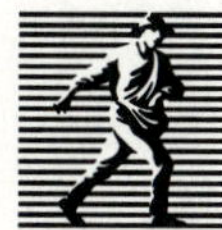

Prentice Hall
Englewood Cliffs, New Jersey 07632

Library of Congress Cataloging-in-Publication Data

Leonard, William L.
Self-study exercises in radiography / William L. Leonard.
p. cm.
Includes bibliographical references.
ISBN 0-13-011651-3
1. Radiography, Medical--Problems, exercises, etc. I. Title.
[DNLM: 1. Technology, Radiologic--examination questions. WN 18
L581s 1995]
RC78.15.L47 1995
616.07'572'076--dc20
DNLM/DLC 94-40511
for Library of Congress CIP

Editorial/Production Supervision and Interior Design: *Cathy O'Connell*
Brady Production Manager: *Pat Walsh*
Director of Production/Manufacturing: *Bruce Johnson*
Prepress/Manufacturing Buyer: *Ilene Sanford*
Acquisitions Editor: *Barbara Krawiec*
Editorial Assistant: *Louise Fullam*
Cover Photography: *©Biophoto Associates/Science Source*
Cover Design: *Wendy Helft, Design W Inc.*
Printer/Binder: *Banta Printers*

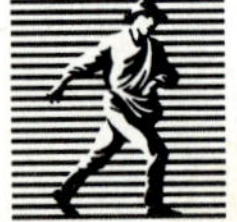

Printed in the United States of America

10 9 8 7 6 5 4 3 2 1

ISBN 0-13-011651-3

PRENTICE-HALL INTERNATIONAL (UK) LIMITED, *London*
PRENTICE-HALL OF AUSTRALIA PTY. LIMITED, *Sydney*
PRENTICE-HALL CANADA INC., *Toronto*
PRENTICE-HALL HISPANOAMERICANA, S.A., *Mexico*
PRENTICE-HALL OF INDIA PRIVATE LIMITED, *New Delhi*
PRENTICE-HALL OF JAPAN, INC., *Tokyo*
SIMON & SCHUSTER ASIA PTE. LTD., *Singapore*
EDITORA PRENTICE-HALL DO BRASIL, LTDA., *Rio de Janeiro*

To My Family
Jo-Carol, Eric, Christina, and Max

Contents

Preface

The radiologic sciences are experiencing tremendous growth, and today's practitioner is required to assume additional responsibilities by possessing a higher degree of technical competence. These rapid changes underscore the need for a stronger base of knowledge to practice effectively in newer modalities. These study modules evolved from a concept first discussed by radiography students in the training program at Bergen Community College. The students were looking for a method to reinforce basic factual information and in turn assist them in preparing for various examinations administered throughout the program.

I have utilized these modules after the student has read the appropriate chapter in the textbook and was presented the materials in a formal lecture class. They can be employed effectively in various intervals of a competency-based education system. The modules have been used for the past two years with numerous contributions and modifications by both students and faculty. Strong positive feedback was presented by our graduates preparing for ARRT Certification. First- and second-year students found them most valuable in assessing their reading and lecture class comprehension.

Instructors can freely select modules that reflect their own unit objectives or weekly lesson plans, prior to actual testing. The modules are not used as a graded exercise but rather as a supplement to lecture, laboratory, and clinical information. These are by no means a shortcut to learning nor are they intended to replace the traditional methods of teaching and learning radiography.

Since most of the information covered in radiography is based on a knowledge or recall level of thinking, these modules can set the foundation necessary for higher levels of cognitive ability. The material for the modules was extracted from 33 of the most commonly used textbooks in radiography, and reflects current ARRT content specifications. The reader will note that the back page of each module contains a foldover answer key and a note section for each item that may require additional information or clarification.

The format corresponds to the five sections covered on the ARRT Certification examination and emphasizes major topics outlined in the ASRT Curriculum Guide in Radiography. I wish you success in your future endeavors in the exciting field of diagnostic radiography.

William L. Leonard RT(R)

Acknowledgments

I wish to commend my lovely wife, Jo-Carol, for her patience and support in the preparation of this manuscript.

Also, I wish to express my sincere appreciation to a very special friend, Mrs. Cindy Klingner, Allied Health and Physical Education Division Executive Secretary, Bergen Community College, for sharing her time and computer expertise with me in the preparation of this book.

The line drawings were contributed by my good friend and colleague, Mr. William F. Toeppe, RT, Manager of Diagnostic Imaging, Bergen Pines County Hospital, Paramus, New Jersey. His high-quality drawings greatly enhanced this manuscript.

My gratitude is also extended to one of my former students, Mrs. Susan Sisti, RT, (R), (M), adjunct clinical instructor, Bergen Community College, for her contribution of modules in mammographic techniques. Her valuable comments and computer skills were most helpful.

Section 1
Radiation Protection

Exercise 1-1 Radiation Protection Terms

DIRECTIONS: Use each answer only once.

A. Latent
B. Instant cell death
C. Highly differentiated cells
D. Leukemogenesis
E. Homeostasis
F. Lipids
G. Inverse square law
H. Linear energy transfer
I. Lysosomes
J. Interphase
K. Lymphocyte
L. Ions
M. Mean energy
N. Hemoglobin
O. Manifest illness
P. Granule
Q. Kinetic
R. Involuntary
S. Hemorrhage
T. Metaphase
U. Leukocytes
V. Incident photon
W. Meiosis
X. Ionization
Y. Key molecule

_____ 1. Conversion of atom to ions
_____ 2. Incoming photon
_____ 3. White blood cells
_____ 4. Oxygen-carrying pigment of red blood cells
_____ 5. Energy of motion
_____ 6. Average energy of x-ray beam
_____ 7. Period following the prodomal stage of acute radiation syndrome
_____ 8. Abnormal escape of blood
_____ 9. Production or origin of leukemia
_____ 10. Insoluble nonmembranous particles found in the cytoplasm
_____ 11. Stores energy for body for a long period of time
_____ 12. Intensity inversely proportional to square of distance
_____ 13. Equilibrium; maintaining normal functions
_____ 14. Amount of radiant energy transferred to an irradiated object per length of travel
_____ 15. Immediate death of a cell from 1000 gray (Gy)
_____ 16. Small pealike sacs containing digestive enzyme
_____ 17. Positively and negatively charged particles
_____ 18. Mature or more specialized cells
_____ 19. White blood cell (WBC): plays active role in producing immunity
_____ 20. Stage of acute syndrome: symptoms are visible
_____ 21. Cell growth that occurs prior to cell division
_____ 22. Genetic cell division reducing chromosomes
_____ 23. Motion caused by muscles not under voluntary control
_____ 24. Maintains normal cell function for survival
_____ 25. Phase of cell division where mitotic spindle is completed

Answer Key	Notes
1. X	
2. V	
3. U	
4. N	
5. Q	
6. M	
7. A	
8. S	
9. D	
10. P	
11. F	
12. G	
13. E	
14. H	
15. B	
16. I	
17. L	
18. C	
19. K	
20. O	
21. J	
22. W	
23. R	
24. Y	
25. T	

Exercise 1-2 Radiation Protection Terms

DIRECTIONS: Use each answer only once.

A. Mitochondria
B. Newton
C. Myeloblasts
D. Milliseivert
E. Nucleic acids
F. Neutron
G. Off focus or stem radiation
H. Mutagens
I. Prodrome
J. Thymine
K. Recessive mutation
L. Milligray
M. Oogonium
N. Neutrophil
O. Mutations
P. Point mutation
Q. Mitosis
R. Nucleus
S. Negatron
T. Mitotic delay
U. Protoplasm
V. Mitotic death
W. Platelets
X. Organogenesis
Y. Positron

_____ 1. Changes in genes
_____ 2. Female germ cell
_____ 3. Circular or oval discs found in blood
_____ 4. Pyrimidine base found only in DNA
_____ 5. White blood stem cells
_____ 6. Chromosome not broken but DNA within is damaged
_____ 7. Gestation from 2 to 6 weeks following conception
_____ 8. $\frac{1}{1000}$ seivert (Sv)
_____ 9. Center of cell containing DNA
_____ 10. Ordinary electron that has a negative charge
_____ 11. Failure of cell to start dividing on time
_____ 12. X-rays from area other than the focal spot
_____ 13. Electrically neutral particle
_____ 14. $\frac{1}{1000}$ Gy
_____ 15. Large, complex macromolecules made up of nucleotides
_____ 16. Cell death occurring after one or more divisions
_____ 17. Unstable, positively charged electron
_____ 18. Functions as the "powerhouse" of the cell
_____ 19. First stage of acute radiation sickness
_____ 20. Agents that increase the frequency of occurrence of mutation
_____ 21. Unit of force
_____ 22. Cell division wherein a parent cell divides to form two daughter cells
_____ 23. Genetic mutation probably not expressed for many generations
_____ 24. Building material of all living cells
_____ 25. Type of leukocyte that helps fight infection

Answer Key	Notes
1. O	
2. M	
3. W	
4. J	
5. C	
6. P	
7. X	
8. D	
9. R	
10. S	
11. T	
12. G	
13. F	
14. L	
15. E	
16. V	
17. Y	
18. A	
19. I	
20. H	
21. B	
22. Q	
23. K	
24. U	
25. N	

Exercise 1-3 Radiation Protection Terms

DIRECTIONS: Use each answer only once.

A. Spermatogonium
B. SID
C. Simple scatter
D. Seivert
E. Undifferentiated
F. Somatic
G. Volt
H. Thymus gland
I. Remnant
J. Hypoxic
K. Short-term somatic effects
L. Victoreen
M. RNA
N. Telophase
O. Electrolytes
P. Thyroid gland
Q. Reproductive cell
R. Unmodified scattering
S. Threshold
T. Skin erythema dose
U. Thrombocytes
V. Voluntary
W. Stem cells
X. Visual acuity
Y. Shadow

_____ 1. Immature or precursor cells
_____ 2. Equal to 1 joule per kilogram
_____ 3. Primary organ of lymphatic system located in the mediastinum
_____ 4. Change appears within minutes, days, or hours
_____ 5. Ability to visualize small image
_____ 6. Point when response to stimulation first occurs
_____ 7. Type of nucleic acid: carries genetic information
_____ 8. About 2 Gy of exposure, causing redness
_____ 9. Immature or nonspecialized cells
_____ 10. Male and female germ cells
_____ 11. Phase of mitosis where second new daughter cells are formed
_____ 12. Type of reproductive organ shield
_____ 13. Chemical compound from acid–base reaction
_____ 14. Initiate blood clotting and prevent hemorrhage
_____ 15. Cells that lack adequate amounts of oxygen
_____ 16. Radiation that reaches the film
_____ 17. Male germ cell
_____ 18. Motion controlled by will
_____ 19. All human body cells except germ
_____ 20. Coherent scattering
_____ 21. Gland in neck that regulates metabolic rate
_____ 22. Gas-filled radiation survey instrument
_____ 23. Source-to-image (receptor) distance
_____ 24. Classical scattering
_____ 25. SI unit of potential difference

Answer Key	Notes
1. W	
2. D	
3. H	
4. K	
5. X	
6. S	
7. M	
8. T	
9. E	
10. Q	
11. N	
12. Y	
13. O	
14. U	
15. J	
16. I	
17. A	
18. V	
19. F	
20. R	
21. P	
22. L	
23. B	
24. C	
25. G	

Exercise 1-4 Radiation Protection Terms

DIRECTIONS: Use each answer only once.

A. Lymphocyte.
B Anaphase
C. Transluminescent dosimeter (TLD)
D. Isotropic
E. Nucleons
F. Linear energy transfer (LET)
G. Curie
H. Latent period
I. 100 mR/yr
J. Compton
K. Hydrogen
L. Dally
M. Bowtie.
N Nausea
O. Gastrointestinal syndrome
P. Radiosensitizers
Q. International Council on Radiation Protection (ICRP)
R. "Cutie Pie"
S. Long-term somatic
T. Hematologic
U. Half-value layer (HVL)
V. National Council on Radiation Protection (NCRP)
W. Carcinogenesis
X. Methotrexate
Y. Monoenergetic

_____ 1. Caused by radiation dose of 150 rem
_____ 2. Useful survey instrument when level exceeds 1 mR/hr
_____ 3. Maximum permissible dose (MPD) for radiographers less than 18 years of age
_____ 4. Particles, protons, and neutrons within the nucleus
_____ 5. Special filters used in computerized tomographic (CT) scanners to compensate body size
_____ 6. Appear after a period of months or years
_____ 7. Duplicate centromeres migrate in opposite direction
_____ 8. Responsible for the most scattered radiation
_____ 9. Regulatory agency that suggested the 10-day rule
_____ 10. Used for stationary area monitoring
_____ 11. Measures the quantity of radioactive material
_____ 12. X-ray emitted at equal energy in all directions
_____ 13. What no sign of radiation sickness is termed to be
_____ 14. Radiosensitizer that enhances the effects of radiation
_____ 15. One tenth-value layer (TVL) is equal to 3.3
_____ 16. Measurement of the rate energy that is transferred to soft tissue
_____ 17. Syndrome produced with a dosage of 200 to 1000 rad
_____ 18. Cell with the highest radiation sensitivity
_____ 19. X-ray beam of a single energy
_____ 20. Radiation doses from 600 to 1000 rad
_____ 21. Agency that put forth the ALARA concept
_____ 22. First American to die from radiation
_____ 23. Chemicals that enhance the effects of radiation
_____ 24. Makes up 60% of the body
_____ 25. Not a form of the acute radiation syndrome

Answer Key	Notes
1. N	
2. R	
3. I	
4. E	
5. M	
6. S	
7. B	
8. J	
9. Q	
10. C	
11. G	
12. D	
13. H	
14. X	
15. U	
16. F	
17. T	
18. A	
19. Y	
20. O	
21. V	
22. L	
23. P	
24. K	
25. W	

Exercise 1-5 Radiation Protection Terms

DIRECTIONS: Use each answer only once.

A. Glandular dose
B. Contact shield
C. Genetically significant dose (GSD)
D. 1 month
E. Bone marrow dose
F. Cardinal rules
G. Extremity monitors
H. Entrance exposure
I. 5 min
J. 66%
K. Gonadal dose
L. 3 months
M. 1.8 m
N. Pocket ionization
O. TLD
P. Certified health physicist (CHP)
Q. Film badge
R. Rayleigh
S. Aluminum and copper
T. ALARA
U. 95% of exposure
V. 88%
W. Control booth
X. Lithium fluoride
Y. Shadow shield

_____ 1. Type of monitor to measure 0 to 200 mR
_____ 2. Unable to measure dosage below 10 mR
_____ 3. Used to determine radiation-induced leukemia
_____ 4. Guideline for lowest possible dose
_____ 5. Known as "skin" or "patient" dose
_____ 6. Shield positioned directly on the patient
_____ 7. Radiation dose to population gene pool
_____ 8. Suspected genetic response dose
_____ 9. Radiation dose occurring during mammography
_____ 10 After film badge, measurement device most often employed
_____ 11. Filters used in film badges
_____ 12. Fluoroscopy, specials, and portables
_____ 13. Also known as coherent scattering
_____ 14. Length of portable exposure cord
_____ 15. Considered a secondary barrier
_____ 16. TLD crystal chip
_____ 17. Time, distance, and shielding
_____ 18. X-ray attenuation from a 0.25mm apron at 75 kVp
_____ 19. Average length of time film badge is worn
_____ 20. Qualified radiation expert abbreviation
_____ 21. Fluoroscopic time limit
_____ 22. Utilized during fluoroscopic and nuclear procedures
_____ 23. Length of time TLD is worn
_____ 24. Lead disc that covers without contact
_____ 25. X-ray attenuation of a 0.5mm Pb apron at 75 kVp

Answer Key	Notes
1. N	
2. O	
3. E	
4. T	
5. H	
6. B	
7. C	
8. K	
9. A	
10. Q	
11. S	
12. U	
13. R	
14. M	
15. W	
16. X	
17. F	
18. J	
19. D	
20. P	
21. I	
22. G	
23. L	
24. Y	
25. V	

Exercise **1-6**

Radiation Protection Standards and Dosages

A. 10 (m rad)
B. 20 (m rad)
C. 25 (m rad)
D. 50 (m rad)
E. 80 (m rad)
F. 100 (m rad)
G. 300 (m radM RAD)
H. 400 (m rad)
I. 1.5-mm al
J. 0.5-mm Al
K. 0.15-mm pb
L. 38 cm
M. 0.25-mm pb
N. 100 mR/hr
O. 2-mm pb
P. 2.5-mm al
Q. 10 R/min
R. 0.1%
S. 2%
T. 30 cm
U. 0.4-mm Pb

DIRECTIONS: For items 1 to 10, estimate the bone marrow dose. Use choices A–H. Answers may be used more than once.

_____ 1. Gallbladder
_____ 2. Lumbar spine
_____ 3. Full-mouth dental
_____ 4. Intravenous pyelogram and gastrointestinal series
_____ 5. Abdomen
_____ 6. Extremity
_____ 7. Cervical spine
_____ 8. Chest
_____ 9. Skull
_____ 10. Pelvis

DIRECTIONS: For items 11 to 24, assign the correct quantity. Use choices I–U. Answers may be used more than once.

_____ 11. Tube housing leakage level
_____ 12. Bucky slot cover thickness
_____ 13. Total filtration for machine above 70 kV
_____ 14. Total filtration of fluoroscope
_____ 15. Source to tabletop (TT) distance on stationary fluoroscope
_____ 16. Protective curtain thickness
_____ 17. Total filtration of machine below 50 kV
_____ 18. Accuracy level of Positive Beam Limitation (PBL) of the SID
_____ 19. Source-to-TT distance on mobile fluoroscope
_____ 20. Intensity during fluoroscope level
_____ 21. Total filtration of machine between 50 and 70 kV
_____ 22. Intensity of scatter 1 m from the patient
_____ 23. Primary protective barrier thickness
_____ 24. Secondary barrier thickness

Answer Key	Notes
1. G	
2. H	
3. C	
4. H	
5. E	
6. A	
7. B	
8. A	
9. D	
10. F	
11. N	
12. M	
13. P	
14. P	
15. L	
16. K	
17. J	
18. S	
19. T	
20. Q	
21. I	
22. R	
23. O	
24. U	

Exercise 1-7 Radiation Protection Dosages

A. Transection
B. Growth arrest
C. Atrophy
D. Necrosis
E. Nephrosclerosis
F. Hypolasia
G. Cataracts
H. Fibrosis
I. Erythema
J. Ascites
K. Ulcers
L. High radiosensitivity
M. Intermediate radiosensitivity
N. Low Radiosensitivity

DIRECTIONS: In items 1 to 12, assign the proper dosage effect. Use choices A–K. Answers may be used more than once.

_____ 1. 1000 to 5000 rad to gastrointestinal tract causes
_____ 2. 200 to 1000 rad to bone marrow causes
_____ 3. 1000 to 5000 rad to liver causes
_____ 4. 1000 to 5000 rad to skin causes
_____ 5. Above 5000 rad to spinal cord causes
_____ 6. 200 to 1000 rad to lymphoid tissue causes
_____ 7. Above 5000 rad to brain causes
_____ 8. 1000 to 5000 rad to growing bone causes
_____ 9. 200 to 1000 rad to gonad causes
_____ 10. Above 5000 rad to muscle causes
_____ 11. 1000 to 5000 rad to kidney causes
_____ 12. 1000 to 5000 rad to cornea causes

DIRECTIONS: In items 13 to 23, match the proper radiosensitivity level to each cell line. Use choices L, M, or N. Answers may be used more than once.

_____ 13. Spermatids
_____ 14. Erythroblasts
_____ 15. Muscle cells
_____ 16. Osteoblasts
_____ 17. Lymphocytes
_____ 18. Chondrocytes
_____ 19. Spermatogonia
_____ 20. Nerve cells
_____ 21. Intestinal crypt cells
_____ 22. Fibroblasts
_____ 23. Endothelial cells

Answer Key	Notes
1. K	
2. F	
3. J	
4. I	
5. A	
6. C	
7. D	
8. B	
9. C	
10. H	
11. E	
12. G	
13. M	
14. L	
15. N	
16. M	
17. L	
18. N	
19. L	
20. N	
21. L	
22. M	
23. M	

Exercise 1-8 Radiobiology Terms

DIRECTIONS: Use each answer only once.

A. Instant death
B. Reproductive death
C. Interphase death
D. Mitotic death
E. Chromosome breakage
F. ALARA
G. Acute radiation syndrome
H. Erythroblasts
I. Absorbed dose
J. Genes
K. Chromosomes
L. Gastrointestinal syndrome
M. Anaphase
N. Genetic damage
O. Epilation
P. Anion
Q. Dose
R. Erg
S. Cytoplasm
T. Free radicals
U. Electrons
V. Germ cells
W. "Cutie pie"
X. Erythrocytes
Y. Granulocyte

_____ 1. Negatively charged atomic particles
_____ 2. Protoplasm that exists outside cells nucleus
_____ 3. Red blood cells
_____ 4. Radiation damage to generations unborn
_____ 5. Occurs to cell at dosages of 1000 Gy
_____ 6. Very reactive chemical molecules with unpaired electrons
_____ 7. Reproductive cells
_____ 8. Amount of energy transferred from ionizing radiation
_____ 9. Leukocyte that fights bacteria
_____ 10. Occurs to cell at dosage of 100 to 1000 rad
_____ 11. Unit of energy and work
_____ 12. Basic units of heredity
_____ 13. Occurs when a cell is irradiated and dies without division
_____ 14. Phase of mitosis where two chromosomes repel each other
_____ 15. Modern guidelines for MPD
_____ 16. Effects cell division adversely: retards or inhibits
_____ 17. Red blood stem cells
_____ 18. Radiation sickness in humans who receive more than 100 rem
_____ 19. Amount of radiant energy absorbed by object
_____ 20. Ionizing radiation interacting directly with DNA molecules
_____ 21. Ionization chamber: type of survey meter
_____ 22. Negatively charged ion
_____ 23. Acute radiation syndrome appears at dose of 1 Gy
_____ 24. Small, rod-shaped bodies; contain genes
_____ 25. Loss of hair

Answer Key	Notes
1. U	
2. S	
3. X	
4. N	
5. A	
6. T	
7. V	
8. I	
9. Y	
10. B	
11. R	
12. J	
13. C	
14. M	
15. F	
16. D	
17. H	
18. G	
19. Q	
20. E	
21. W	
22. P	
23. L	
24. K	
25. 0	

Exercise 1-9 Radiobiology

A. High sensitivity
B. Intermediate sensitivity
C. Low sensitivity
D. 5000 mR/yr
E. 500 mR
F. 100 mR
G. 15 rem/yr
H. 75 rem/yr
I. 30 rem/yr
J. 0.17 rem/yr
K. 1 rad
L. 250 mGy
M. 25 rem
N. 450 rem
O. 600 rem

DIRECTIONS: In items 1 to 12, match the proper sensitivity level to each body part. Use choices A, B, or C. Answers may be used more than once.

_____ 1. Muscle
_____ 2. Cornea
_____ 3. Gonads
_____ 4. Brain
_____ 5. Liver and thyroid
_____ 6. Lymphoid tissue
_____ 7. Growing bone
_____ 8. Kidney
_____ 9. Spinal cord
_____ 10. Bone marrow
_____ 11. Gastrointestinal tract
_____ 12. Skin

DIRECTIONS: In items 13 to 24, assign the correct quantity. Use choices D–O. Answers may be used more than once.

_____ 13. Same as 10 mGy
_____ 14. Causes blood changes
_____ 15. MPD for hands
_____ 16. Recommended MPD during gestation
_____ 17. Lethal dose (LD) $^{50}/_{30}$ dosage
_____ 18. MPD for radiographer less than 18 years of age
_____ 19. Dosage may justify therapeutic abortion
_____ 20. Yearly occupational MPD
_____ 21. MPD for skin
_____ 22. MPD for forearms
_____ 23. Fatal dosage for humans
_____ 24. MPD for general population

Answer Key

1. C
2. B
3. A
4. C
5. B
6. A
7. B
8. B
9. C
10. A
11. B
12. B
13. K
14. M
15. H
16. E
17. N
18. F
19. L
20. D
21. G
22. I
23. O
24. J

Notes

Exercise 1-10 Formulas and Laws

DIRECTIONS: Use each answer only once.

A. Electrostatics
B. HVL
C. Characteristic Curve
D. Ohm's law
E. Laws
F. Transformer
G. Inverse square
H. Lenz's law
I. Time and temperature
J. Radioactive decay
K. Grid ratio
L. 15% rule
M. Conservation
N. Line focus principle
O. Motor
P. Reciprocity
Q. Attenuation
R. Bergonié–Tribondeau law
S. mAs and distance
T. Tube rating chart
U. Magnetism
V. Intensification factor
W. Magnetic
X. Caliper adjustment
Y. Laws of motion

_____ 1. Formula dealing with half-life
_____ 2. Gives guidelines for safe tube operation
_____ 3. Direction that induced current would flow
_____ 4. Relationship of intensity to distance
_____ 5. Radiosensitivity was a function of metabolic state of tissue radiated
_____ 6. Alternation in density by adjusting kV
_____ 7. Plots various densities on graph
_____ 8. For every centimeter, go +2 kV
_____ 9. Focus smaller when projected toward film
_____ 10. Formula required to maintain density when changing distance
_____ 11. Likes repel and unlikes attract
_____ 12. Intensity × exposure duration
_____ 13. Observations based on human experience
_____ 14. Every 2 degrees is ± ½ min
_____ 15. Height of lead strips to distance between
_____ 16 Five laws governing static electricity
_____ 17. Amount of filtration to cut beam in half
_____ 18. Body will remain at rest unless acted on by force
_____ 19. Right hand if thumb and first two fingers are at right angles
_____ 20. Volts = amperes × current
_____ 21. Energy cannot be created or destroyed
_____ 22. Number of turns in secondary to number of turns in primary
_____ 23. Relationship: density from nonscreen to screens
_____ 24. Force of attraction or repulsion inversely proportional to the square of distance
_____ 25. Every millimeter of filtration removes about 4 kV

Answer Key

1. J
2. T
3. H
4. G
5. R
6. L
7. C
8. X
9. N
10. S
11. U
12. P
13. E
14. I
15. K
16. A
17. B
18. Y
19. O
20. D
21. M
22. F
23. V
24. W
25. Q

Notes

Section 2
Equipment Operation and Maintenance

Exercise 2-1 Equipment Operation and Maintenance

DIRECTIONS: Use each answer only once.

A. Tryristor
B. Extra focal
C. Vidicon
D. PBL
E. Line-voltage compensator
F. Circuit breaker
G. Turns ratio
H. Electronic
I. Brightness gain
J. K-shell absorption edge
K. Induction
L. Thermal energy
M. Signal
N. Effective
O. Impulse
P. Proportional counter
Q. Rayleigh
R. Microfocus
S. Backup timer
T. Window
U. Mechanical
V. Solenoid
W. Fulgrum
X. Hysteresis
Y. Noise

_____ 1. Point where primary x-ray beam exits the tube
_____ 2. Coherent scattering can be Thompson or
_____ 3. Detection instrument that measures alpha and beta radiation
_____ 4. 99% or more of kinetic energy of projectile electrons is converted to
_____ 5. Focal spot projected onto patient and film
_____ 6. Simple spring-wound timing devices
_____ 7. Motor that drives the rotating anode
_____ 8. Special tubes used in macroradiographs
_____ 9. Protects the patient from overexposure when using an (AEC)
_____ 10. TV camera tube most often used in fluoroscopy
_____ 11. Lagging loss from continually changing alternating current (AC)
_____ 12. Device that keeps incoming voltage constant
_____ 13. Looped coil with current flowing through
_____ 14. Mimification factor × flux gain =
_____ 15. Timer used for exposures as short as 0.001 sec
_____ 16. Occurs when x-ray energy is equal to binding energy
_____ 17. Number of secondary windings to primary windings
_____ 18. Electromagnet that protects from an overload
_____ 19. Silicon-controlled rectifier
_____ 20. Automatically collimates to the film size
_____ 21. Imaginary pivot point about which the tube and film move
_____ 22. Off-focus radiation not produced at focal spot
_____ 23. Also known as "background electricity"
_____ 24. Timer that counts the number of sine-wave pulses
_____ 25. Electric current that conveys a message

Answer Key	Notes
1. T	
2. Q	
3. P	
4. L	
5. N	
6. U	
7. K	
8. R	
9. S	
10. C	
11. X	
12. E	
13. V	
14. I	
15. H	
16. J	
17. G	
18. F	
19. A	
20. D	
21. W	
22. B	
23. Y	
24. O	
25. M	

Exercise 2-2 Accessory Equipment

DIRECTIONS: Use each answer only once.

A. Resolution bar pattern
B. Compression device
C. Positive beam limitation
D. Trough filter
E. Phototimer or mAs timer
F. Penetrometer
G. Hurter and Driffield curve
H. Lead mats
I. Filter
J. Digital
K. Aperture diaphragm
L. Circuit breaker
M. Image receptor
N. Tube rating chart
O. Wire mesh
P. Electroscope
Q. Densitometer
R. Vignetting
S. Pocket ionization chamber
T. Spinning top
U. Control grid
V. Pinhole camera
W. "Cutie pie"
X. Face plate
Y. Rate meter

_____ 1. Battery-operated radiation meter
_____ 2. Absorbs soft rays and reduces skin dosage
_____ 3. Plots relationship of density and exposure
_____ 4. Records image on film
_____ 5. Measures density levels for calibration
_____ 6. X-rays forming an electronic image
_____ 7. Penlike radiation monitor
_____ 8. Utilized to record film sharpness
_____ 9. Reduction of brightness around the periphery
_____ 10. Measure quantity of radiation reaching the film
_____ 11. Outer layer or window of a television camera
_____ 12. Stepwedge used to measure penetration
_____ 13. Measures the presence of electric charge
_____ 14. Used to measure effective focal spot size
_____ 15. Placed on tabletop to absorb scatter radiation
_____ 16. Electromagnet that prevents overloading
_____ 17. Used to retain contrast media in the kidney
_____ 18. Utilized to check rectification and timing circuit
_____ 19. Averages the rate of pulses
_____ 20. Changes field size close to tube housing
_____ 21. Measures safe exposure levels
_____ 22. Automated device that controls field size
_____ 23. Double-wedge filter
_____ 24. Attached to the electron gun to control intensity
_____ 25. Placed on cassette to measure film screen contact

Answer Key	Notes
1. W	
2. I	
3. G	
4. M	
5. Q	
6. J	
7. S	
8. A	
9. R	
10. E	
11. X	
12. F	
13. P	
14. V	
15. H	
16. L	
17. B	
18. T	
19. Y	
20. Y	
21. K	
22. C	
23. D	
24. U	
25. O	

Exercise 2-3 Electricity and Magnetism

DIRECTIONS: Use each answer only once.

A. Volt
B. Ammeter
C. Series
D. Battery
E. Rheostat
F. Insulator
G. Electromotive force (EMF)
H. Resistor
I. Electrodynamics
J. Direct current
K. Four-valve tubes
L. Ampere
M. Watts
N. Transformer
O. Silicon
P. Voltmeter
Q. Magnetic
R. Electrostatics
S. Conductor
T. Capacitor
U. Class
V. Ohm
W. Niobium
X. Alternating current
Y. Copper

_____ 1. Inhibits the flow of electrons
_____ 2. Electrons oscillating back and forth
_____ 3. Stores electric charges
_____ 4. Has ability to attract iron
_____ 5. Study of fixed or stationary electric charges
_____ 6. Electrons flowing in one direction
_____ 7. Semiconductive material
_____ 8. All circuit elements are connected in a line
_____ 9. Increases or decreases voltage
_____ 10. Unit of measurement of electric power
_____ 11. Superconductive material
_____ 12. Measures electric current
_____ 13. Conductive material
_____ 14. Substance that allows free electron flow
_____ 15. Known as a variable resistor
_____ 16. Unit of electrical resistance
_____ 17. Required for full-wave rectification
_____ 18. Unit of electrical potential
_____ 19. Inhibits flow of electrons
_____ 20. Also known as "electric potential"
_____ 21. Measures electric potential
_____ 22. Unit of electrical current
_____ 23. Provides electric potential
_____ 24. Insulative material
_____ 25. Study of electrostatic charges in motion

Answer Key

Notes

1. F
2. X
3. T
4. Q
5. R
6. J
7. O
8. C
9. N
10. M
11. W
12. B
13. Y
14. S
15. E
16. V
17. K
18. A
19. H
20. G
21. P
22. L
23. D
24. U
25. I

Exercise 2-4 X-Ray Production

DIRECTIONS: Use each answer only once.

A. Quality
B. Space-charge effect
C. Pair production
D. Inner-shell electrons
E. Dead man
F. Attenuation
G. $2N^2$
H. Radiopaque
I. Bremsstrahlung
J. PBL
K. Photoelectric
L. Quantity
M. Backscatter
N. K shell
O. +15% kVp
P. HVL
Q. Characteristic
R. Cone cutting
S. Filtration
T. Low kV
U. L shell
V. Trough filter
W. Compton
X. Differential absorption
Y. Radiolucent

_____ 1. Results in high x-ray absorption
_____ 2. Photons scattered back in the direction of the incident beam
_____ 3. Characteristic of making of a radiograph
_____ 4. Photon absorption interaction
_____ 5. Negative charges that form a cloud around the filament
_____ 6. Braking of projectile electron by nucleus
_____ 7. Compensates for differences in subject radiopacity
_____ 8. Recoil electron
_____ 9. Increases effective energy of the beam
_____ 10. Produces soft-tissue images
_____ 11. Interaction is sufficiently violent to ionize the target atom
_____ 12. Automatic positive beam-limiting device
_____ 13. Holds eight electrons
_____ 14. Reduction in number of x-rays at beam
_____ 15. Greater binding energy
_____ 16. Occurs at 1.02-MeV levels of energy
_____ 17. Relates to beam's energy (kV)
_____ 18. Holds two electrons
_____ 19. X-rays pass through easily
_____ 20. Type of switch required for fluoroscopic exposure
_____ 21. Formula to calculate number of electrons in each shell
_____ 22. Unexposed edge of cone interferes with beam
_____ 23. Relates to number of electrons (mAs)
_____ 24. Equivalent to doubling the mAs value
_____ 25. Amount of filtration: cuts beam intensity by one-half

Answer Key

Notes

1. H
2. M
3. X
4. K
5. B
6. I
7. V
8. W
9. S
10. T
11. Q
12. J
13. U
14. F
15. D
16. C
17. A
18. N
19. Y
20. E
21. G
22. R
23. L
24. O
25. P

Exercise 2-5 X-Ray Tubes

DIRECTIONS: Use each answer only once.

A. Stator
B. 700:1 or 1000:1
C. 1 to 2% thorium
D. 220 V
E. 100 mR/hr at 1 m
F. Dose equivalent
G. 0.3 to 3 mm
H. 1 mm × 4 mm
I. Anode heel effect
J. Effective focal spot
K. 3400 rpm
L. Electric taps
M. Focusing cup
N. Milliammeter
O. Window
P. AC
Q. 7 cm
R. Heat units
S. 7 to 18 degrees
T. Pulsating DC
U. Rotor
V. Focal spot
W. Tube rating chart
X. Victoreen condenser R meter
Y. Rectifier

_____ 1. Actual target area for a stationary tube
_____ 2. Gas-filled survey instrument used to calibrate x-ray units
_____ 3. Area of target from which x-ray emitted
_____ 4. Condenses electron beam to small area of anode
_____ 5. mas × kV × number of exposures
_____ 6. Diagnostic x-ray tube target angle
_____ 7. Normal rotating anode diameter
_____ 8. Ratio of high-voltage transformer
_____ 9. Primary x-rays emitted through this port
_____ 10. Part located outside the glass envelope
_____ 11. Measures x-ray tube current
_____ 12. Filament coating
_____ 13. Current needed to operate transformers
_____ 14. Effective target area
_____ 15. Plots safe levels of exposure
_____ 16. Acceptable level of leakage at housing
_____ 17. Connections located on the autotransformer
_____ 18. Shaft of copper bars and soft-iron inside tube
_____ 19. Most x-ray machines power source
_____ 20. Speed of most rotating anodes
_____ 21. Current supplied to x-ray tube for exposure
_____ 22. X-ray tube's effective focal spot sizes
_____ 23. Changes ac to pulsating dc
_____ 24. Radiation difference in intensity on cathode and anode side
_____ 25. Absorbed dose × quality factor (QF) =

Answer Key

1. H
2. X
3. V
4. M
5. R
6. S
7. Q
8. B
9. O
10. A
11. N
12. C
13. P
14. J
15. W
16. E
17. L
18. U
19. D
20. K
21. T
22. G
23. Y
24. I
25. F

Notes

Exercise 2-6 X-Ray Tubes

DIRECTIONS: Use each answer only once.

A. 10,000 rpm
B. Thermionic emission
C. Small and large
D. Thorium
E. Tube rating chart
F. 99.8%
G. Bremsstrahlung radiation
H. Lambda
I. Vacuum
J. 10%
K. Tungsten
L. 10 to 12 V, 3 to 5 A
M. 0.1 to 0.5 Å
N. 186,000 miles/sec
O. Tungsten–rhenium steel
P. Remnant
Q. Autotransformer
R. 0.2 to 1.0%
S. 2.5-mm Al
T. mas × kVp × QF
U. 4 kV
V. Molybdenum
W. 40 to 150 kV
X. Leakage
Y. 0.3 to 2.5 mm

_____ 1. Adjusted when kV is changed or selected
_____ 2. Each 1 mm of Al filter approximately
_____ 3. Filtration for tubes operating above 70 kVp
_____ 4. Radiation that does not come out of window
_____ 5. Sizes of dual-focus tube filaments
_____ 6 Condition in tube to allow free flow of electrons
_____ 7. Speed that x-rays travel
_____ 8. Boiling-off of electrons at cathode
_____ 9. Dual filaments
_____ 10. Amount of x-ray produced when electrons hit the target
_____ 11. Speed of high-capacity anodes
_____ 12 Gives cathode more durability
_____ 13. Useful range of diagnostic voltage
_____ 14. Occurs at anode (braking)
_____ 15. Amount of heat generated per exposure
_____ 16. Greek symbol for wavelength
_____ 17. Calculation for heat units
_____ 18. Composition of anode
_____ 19. System to plot safe tube limits
_____ 20. Filament component
_____ 21. Required to make "space cloud"
_____ 22. Useful range of diagnostic x-rays
_____ 23. Focusing cup
_____ 24. Useful radiation that makes image
_____ 25. Amount of scattered radiation

Answer Key

1. Q
2. U
3. S
4. X
5. Y
6. I
7. N
8. B
9. C
10. R
11. A
12. D
13. W
14. G
15. F
16. H
17. T
18. 0
19. E
20. K
21. L
22. M
23. V
24. P
25. J

Notes

Exercise 2-7 X-Ray Circuits

DIRECTIONS: Use each answer only once.

A. Leakage flux
B. Primary
C. Ionization chamber
D. Line voltage
E. 4 to 12
F. Autotransformer
G. Step-up transformer
H. Synchronous timer
I. AC
J. Milliamperes
K. 3 to 5 A
L. Fuses
M. Sievert
N. Timer switch
O. Saturable reactor
P. Secondary
Q. Hysteresis
R. High-voltage transformer
S. Impulse timer
T. Half-wave rectification
U. Three-phase power
V. Prereading kV meter
W. Ripple
X. Amperes
Y. Full-wave rectification

_____ 1. Characterization of voltage waveforms
_____ 2. Compensates for slow line-voltage fluctuations
_____ 3. Measurement of tube current
_____ 4. Used to complete the x-ray exposure
_____ 5. Operates at 1/120 to 1/5 sec
_____ 6. SI unit of absorbed dose equivalent
_____ 7. Low-voltage circuit is also the
_____ 8. Variation of filament current is controlled by the __________
_____ 9. Works in range 1/20 to about 20 sec
_____ 10. Required to beat the filament
_____ 11. High-voltage circuit is also the
_____ 12. Often called the x-ray generator
_____ 13. Special type of AEC control
_____ 14. Puts out a higher voltage than applied
_____ 15. Voltage supplied to the x-ray department
_____ 16. Heat loss of electrical energy
_____ 17. Varies voltage supplied to primary of the transformer
_____ 18. Measurement of filament current
_____ 19. Incoming current supply
_____ 20. Self, or uses one to two-valve tubes
_____ 21. Protects equipment and prevents fire hazard
_____ 22. Four-valve tubes provide
_____ 23. Loss of magnetic charges in the air
_____ 24. Required tube filament voltage
_____ 25. Three simultaneous voltage waveforms

Answer Key	Notes
1. W	
2. V	
3. J	
4. N	
5. S	
6. M	
7. B	
8. O	
9. H	
10. K	
11. P	
12. R	
13. C	
14. G	
15. D	
16. Q	
17. F	
18. X	
19. I	
20. T	
21. L	
22. Y	
23. A	
24. E	
25. U	

Exercise 2-8 Famous Discoverers

DIRECTIONS: Use each answer only once.

A. Galvanti
B. Faraday
C. Joule's law
D. Einstein
E. Maxwell
F. Joule
G. Bucky
H. Stokes
I. Ohm
J. Potter
K. Coolidge
L. Mendeleev
M. Mistretta
N. Becquerel
O. Volta
P. Pupin
Q. Roentgen
R. Rutherford
S. Crookes
T. Morgan
U. Edison
V. Bohr
W. Rankin
X. Curie
Y. Hounsfield

_____ 1. Developed hot-filament x-ray tube
_____ 2. Developed first reciprocating grid
_____ 3. Measured different potential in metals
_____ 4. Demonstrates digital fluoroscopy
_____ 5. Formed the periodic table
_____ 6. Developed first CT scanner
_____ 7. Experimented with atoms and mass
_____ 8. Experimented with dosages of radiation
_____ 9. Stated work = force × distance
_____ 10. Measured various electromagnetic radiations
_____ 11. Mother of radioactivity
_____ 12. Invented first battery
_____ 13. Developed first gas tube with cathode rays
_____ 14. Conducted experiments with wavelength
_____ 15. Conducted experiments with barium platinocyanide
_____ 16. Developed first grid
_____ 17. Developed first intensifying screen
_____ 18. Stated energy is mass × speed of light squared in a vacuum
_____ 19. Conducted experiments with mass, space and atom
_____ 20. Early experimenter with calcium tungstate
_____ 21. Experimented with uranium and radioactive material
_____ 22. Showed relationship between volts, amperes, and resistance
_____ 23. Developed first calcium tungstate screen
_____ 24. First patient to be radiographed
_____ 25. Developed first electronic phototiming device

Answer Key	Notes
1. K	
2. J	
3. A	
4. M	
5. L	
6. Y	
7. R	
8. F	
9. C	
10. B	
11. X	
12. O	
13. S	
14. E	
15. W	
16. G	
17. H	
18. D	
19. V	
20. U	
21. N	
22. I	
23. P	
24. Q	
25. T	

Exercise 2-9 Tube Rating Chart

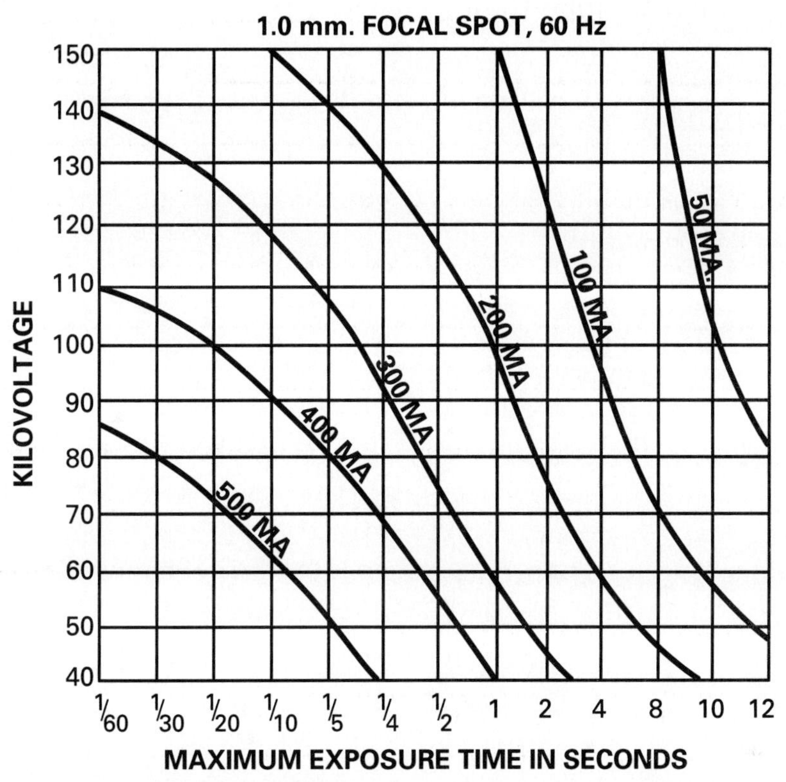

Plate 1 (Artwork courtesy of William F. Toeppe)

Plate 1. Tube Rating Chart

1. What is maximum kV at 400 mA 1/5 sec?________________
2. What is maximum time at 90 kV 200 mA? ________________
3. What is maximum kV at 200 mA 1 sec? ________________
4. What is maximum time at 400 mA 90 kV? ________________
5. What is maximum mA at 1 sec 95 kV? ________________

Plate 1. Tube Rating Chart

1.80 kV
2. 1½ sec
3.98 kV
4. 1⁄10 sec
5.200 mA

Exercise **2-10 Anode Cooling Chart**

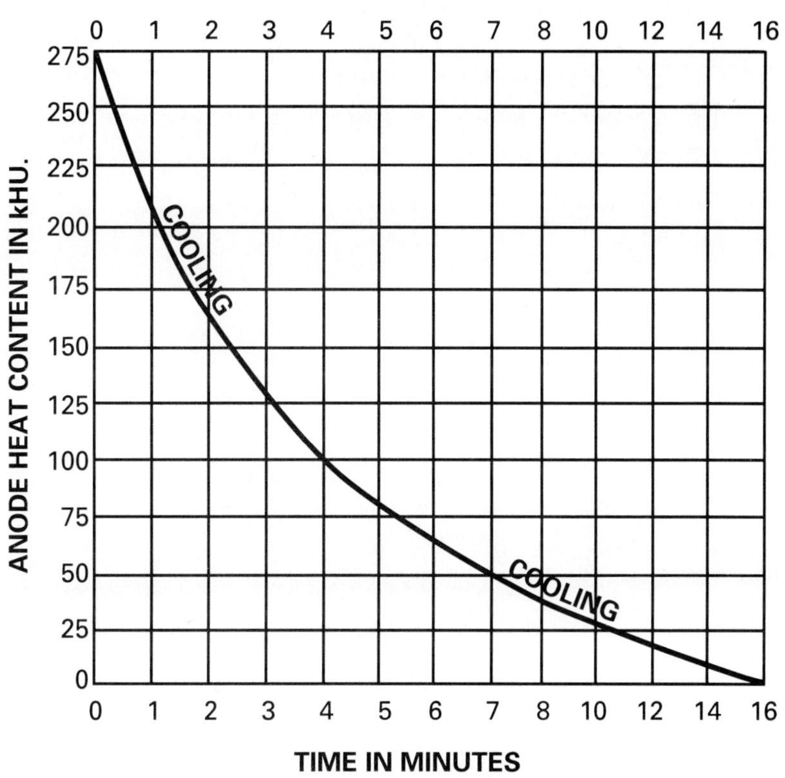

Plate 2 (Artwork courtesy of William F. Toeppe)

Plate 2. Anode Cooling Chart

1. Cooling time required for 175 kHU ____________________
2. Cooling time required for 75 kHU ____________________
3. At 6 min, what is maximum kHU? ____________________

Plate 2. Anode Cooling Chart

1. 16 minutes – 1½ = 14½ minutes
2. 16 minutes minus 5 minutes = 11 minutes
3. 25

Exercise 2-11 X-Ray Tube

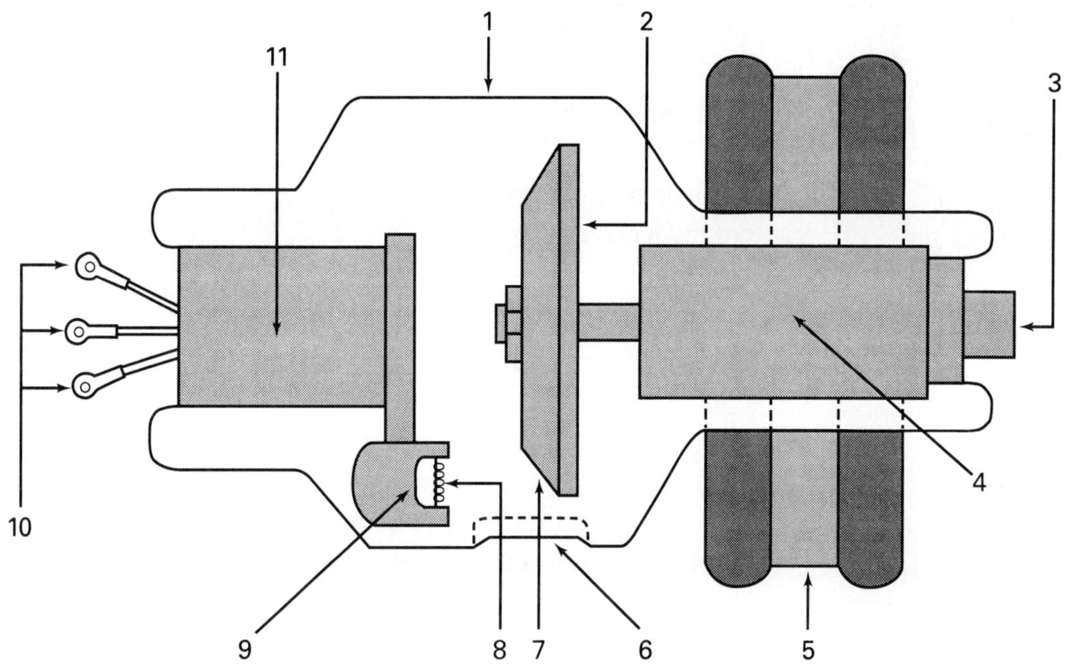

Plate 3 (Artwork courtesy of William F. Toeppe)

Plate 3. X-Ray Tube

Identify the parts of the x-ray tube labeled 1 to 11.

1.
2.
3.
4.
5.
6.
7.
8.
9.
10.
11.

Plate 3. X-Ray Tube

1. Pyrex glass envelope
2. Rotating anode disc
3. Anode
4. Rotor of induction motor
5. Stator of induction motor
6. Glass window
7. Tungsten target
8. Cathode filamen
9. Focusing cup
10. Cathode connections
11. Cathode

Exercise 2-12 X-Ray Circuit

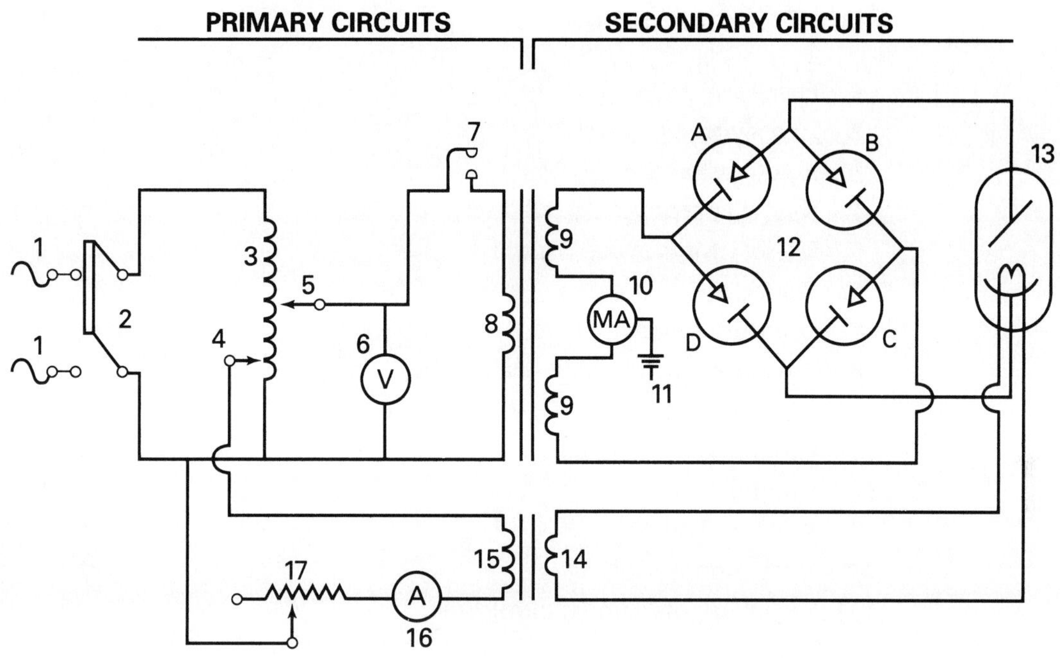

Plate 4 (Artwork courtesy of William F. Toeppe)

Plate 4. X-Ray Circuit

Identify the parts of the x-ray circuit labeled 1 to 17.

1.
2.
3.
4.
5.
6.
7.
8.
9.
10.
11.
12.
13.
14.
15.
16.
17.

Plate 4. X-Ray Circuit

1. Fuses
2. Line switch
3. Autotransformer
4. X-ray filament voltage adjuster
5. KV selector (voltage control)
6. Voltmeter
7. Exposure switch
8. Primary of high-voltage transformer
9. Secondary of high-voltage transformer
10. Grounded milliammeter
11. Ground
12. Rectifier diodes
13. X-ray tube
14. Secondary of filament transformer
15. Primary of filament transformer
16. Filament ammeter
17. Rheostat (milliampere selector)

Section 3
Image Production and Evaluation

Exercise 3-1 Radiographic Density

DIRECTIONS: Without compensation indicate the change, if any, in film quality for each item. Answers may be used more than once.

A. Density increased
B. Density decreased
C. No visible change

_____ 1. Increase from 96 kV to 98 kV
_____ 2. Change from 2in. OFD to 12in. OFD
_____ 3. Change 100 mA small FS to 100 mA large FS
_____ 4. Change from 12:1 grid to 8:1 grid
_____ 5. Increase from 40in. to 50in. SID
_____ 6. Collimate from 14 × 17 field to 8 × 10 field
_____ 7. Change from 80 kV to 92 kV (15% rule)
_____ 8. Increase from 42 kV to 45 kV
_____ 9. Go from 100 mA small FS to 300 mA large FS
_____ 10 Tube 20 degrees increasing Pt absorption
_____ 11. Change from 40in. SID to 24in. SID
_____ 12. Decrease from 72in. SID to 70in. SID
_____ 13. Go from 100 mAs to 200 mAs
_____ 14. Convert to a higher-speed film
_____ 15. Go from medium screen to rare earth screen
_____ 16. Developing temperature off 5 degrees
_____ 17. Change from 12:1 moving grid to no grid
_____ 18. Change from 10:1 grid to 16:1 grid
_____ 19. Change from high-speed cassette to CBH (cardboard holder)
_____ 20. Change from 200 mAs to 225 mAs
_____ 21. Go from 10 × 12 field to 14 × 17 field
_____ 22. Remove 1.5 mm of added filtration
_____ 23. From normal tissue technique to atrophic condition
_____ 24. Change from 8in. OFD to 1in. OFD
_____ 25. Use cassette with poor film–screen contact

Answer Key	Notes
1. C	
2. B	
3. C	
4. A	
5. B	
6. B	
7. A	
8. A	
9. A	
10. B	
11. A	
12. C	
13. A	
14. A	
15. A	
16. C	
17. A	
18. B	
19. B	
20. C	
21. A	
22. A	
23. A	
24. A	
25. C	

Exercise 3-2 Radiographic Contrast

DIRECTIONS: Without compensation, indicate the change, if any, in film quality for each item. Answers may be used more than once.

A. Contrast increased
B. Contrast decreased
C. No visible change

_____ 1. Change from 2in. OFD to 10in. OFD
_____ 2. Change from 100 mA small FS to 100 mA large FS
_____ 3. Go from normal bone technique to atrophic condition
_____ 4. Increase from 70 kV to 72 kV
_____ 5. Change from 12:1 grid to 8:1 grid
_____ 6. Use a cassette with poor film–screen contact
_____ 7. Increase from 70 kV to 80 kV
_____ 8. Go from 100 mAs to 300 mAs
_____ 9. Change from 40in. SID to 20in. SID
_____ 10. Go from 100 mA small FS to 500 mA large FS
_____ 11. Go from 10 × 12 field to beyond 14 × 17 field
_____ 12. Decrease from 92 kV to 80 kV (15% rule)
_____ 13. Change from 6in. OFD to no OFD
_____ 14. Increase SID from 40in. SID to 60in. SID
_____ 15. Convert slow-speed screen to high-speed screen
_____ 16. Automatic processor's temperature and replenishment rate abnormal
_____ 17. Collimate from 14 × 17 field to 8 × 10 field
_____ 18. Use nonscreen film in a high-speed cassette
_____ 19. Decrease from 40in. SID to 36in. SID
_____ 20. Increase from 100 mAs to 120 mAs
_____ 21. Increase from 40 kV to 46 kV
_____ 22. Go from medium (100)-speed screens to CBH
_____ 23. Remove 1.5 mm of added filtration
_____ 24. Tube 15 degrees increasing Pt absorption
_____ 25. Change 12:1 moving grid to 8:1 stationary grid

Answer Key

Notes

1. A
2. C
3. B
4. C
5. B
6. C
7. B
8. B
9. B
10. B
11. B
12. A
13. B
14. A
15. A
16. B
17. A
18. B
19. C
20. C
21. B
22. B
23. C
24. C
25. B

Exercise 3-3 Radiographic Definition

DIRECTIONS: Without compensation, indicate the change, if any, in film quality for each item. Answers may be used more than once.

A. Definition increase

B. Definition decrease

C. No visible change

_____ 1. Go from 14 × 17 field to 8 × 10 field

_____ 2. Change from 92 kVp to 80 kVp (15% rule)

_____ 3. Change from 10:1 grid to 16:1 grid

_____ 4. Increase from 40in. SID to 60in. SID

_____ 5. Increase from 60 kVp to 80 kVp

_____ 6. Go from 2.0-mm focal spot to 0.3-mm focal spot

_____ 7. Go from 100 mAs to 200 mAs

_____ 8. Change from medium-speed screen to CBH

_____ 9. Change from 2in. OFD to 10in. OFD

_____ 10. Convert rare earth screen to slow-speed screen

_____ 11. Use cassette with poor film–screen contact

_____ 12. Change exposure time from 1 sec to 1/10 sec

_____ 13. Change from 100 mA large FS to 100 mA small FS

_____ 14. Remove 1 mm of added filtration

_____ 15. Decrease from 40in. SID to 24in. SID

_____ 16. Increase from 40 kVp to 44 kVp

_____ 17. Change from normal tissue technique to atrophic condition

_____ 18. Change 16:1 rhombic grid to 8:1 focus grid

_____ 19. Angle the tube 20 degrees cephalic

_____ 20. Increase from 100 mAs to 120 mAs

_____ 21. Change from 10in. OFD to 2in. OFD

_____ 22. Automatic processor temperature off 5°

_____ 23. Change from 45-degree tube angle to 5-degree tube angle

_____ 24. Change slow-speed screen to high-speed screen

_____ 25. Change exposure time from ½ sec to 2 sec

Answer Key	Notes
1. A	
2. C	
3. C	
4. A	
5. C	
6. A	
7. C	
8. A	
9. B	
10. A	
11. B	
12. A	
13. A	
14. C	
15. B	
16. C	
17. C	
18. C	
19. B	
20. C	
21. A	
22. C	
23. A	
24. B	
25. B	

Exercise 3-4 Radiographic Magnification and Distortion

DIRECTIONS: Without compensation, indicate the change, if any, in film quality for each item. Answers may be used more than once.

A. Distortion increase
B. Distortion decrease
C. No visible change

_____ 1. Change from 2in. OFD to 12in. OFD
_____ 2. Collimate from 10 × 12 field to 8 × 10 field
_____ 3. Use cassette with an overall poor film–screen contact
_____ 4. Take exposure when patient is moving
_____ 5. Go from normal tissue technique to atrophic condition
_____ 6. Change from rare earth screen to slow-speed screen
_____ 7. Change from 36in. SID to 48in. SID
_____ 8. Increase from 80 kVp to 92 kVp (15% rule)
_____ 9. Increase abdominal exposure time from ¼ sec to 2 sec
_____ 10. Change from a 6:1 grid to a 16:1 grid
_____ 11. Body part not at right angle to central ray
_____ 12. Change from 100-mA small FS to 100-mA large FS
_____ 13. Hand-develop for 5 min at 72 degrees
_____ 14. Go from manual technique to AEC
_____ 15. Use screen film in a CBH
_____ 16. Change from stationary grid to moving grid
_____ 17. Change from hand developing to automatic processor
_____ 18. Central ray not directed to center of film
_____ 19. Increase from 40in. SID to 60in. SID
_____ 20. Change from 6ft SID to 10ft SID
_____ 21. Go from 100 mAs to 300 mAs
_____ 22. Remove 1 mm of added filtration
_____ 23. Angle tube from 5° cephalic to 35° cephalic
_____ 24. Change from 1.5 mm FS to 0.3 mm FS
_____ 25. Radiograph patient semierect with no tube angle

Answer Key

Notes

1. A
2. C
3. A
4. A
5. C
6. C
7. B
8. C
9. A
10. C
11. A
12. C
13. C
14. C
15. C
16. C
17. C
18. A
19. B
20. B
21. C
22. C
23. A
24. C
25. A

Exercise 3-5 Radiographic Quality

DIRECTIONS: Answers may be used more than once. Items can require more than one answer.

A. Affects density
B. Affects contrast
C. Affects definition
D. Affects distortion

_____ 1. Take exposure during patient movement
_____ 2. Change from 72in. SID to 48in. SID
_____ 3. Change to cassette with poor film–screen contact
_____ 4. Change high-speed screen to rare earth screen
_____ 5. Go from 0-degree angle to 35-degree caudad
_____ 6. Utilize a CBH instead of a cassette
_____ 7. Automatic processors: temperature and replenishment rate off
_____ 8. Change kV up 15%
_____ 9. Angle tube 25 degrees with a rhombic grid
_____ 10. Change from grid to tabletop
_____ 11. Normal chest-to-pulmonary edema
_____ 12. Utilize lead mats on tabletop for lateral coccyx
_____ 13. Go from a 2.0-mm focal spot to an 0.3 mm focal spot
_____ 14. Radiograph a patient with ascites
_____ 15. Change from 8 × 10 field to 14 × 17 field
_____ 16. Utilize a 5in. air gap from 0in. OFD
_____ 17. Change from 10 × 12 field to extension cone
_____ 18. Body part not parallel to film
_____ 19. Central ray not directed to body part center
_____ 20. Increase mAs from 100 mAs to 300 mAs
_____ 21. Radiograph a patient with sclerosis
_____ 22. Change from 46 kV to 54 kV
_____ 23. Go from normal bone technique to osteoporosis
_____ 24. Take exposure with off-center grid error
_____ 25. Change from an 8:1 grid to a 12:1 grid

Answer Key	Notes
1. C, D	
2. A, B, C, D	
3. C	
4. A, B, C	
5. A, D	
6. A, B, C	
7. A, B	
8. A, B	
9. A, B, D	
10. A, B	
11. A, B	
12. A, B	
13. C	
14. A, B	
15. A, B, C	
16. A, B, C, D	
17. A, B, C	
18. C, D	
19. D	
20. A, B	
21. A, B	
22. A, B	
23. A, B	
24. A, B, D	
25. A, B	

Exercise 3-6 Pathology and Exposure Factors

DIRECTIONS: Answers may be used more than once.

A. Hard to penetrate
B. Easy to penetrate

_____ 1. Empyema
_____ 2. Active osteomyelitis
_____ 3. Hydropneumothorax
_____ 4. Gout
_____ 5. Pneumonia
_____ 6. Acromegaly
_____ 7. Asceptic necrosis
_____ 8. Atelectasis
_____ 9. Leukemia
_____ 10. Acute Kyphosis
_____ 11. Malignancy of bowel
_____ 12. Paget's disease
_____ 13. Carcinoma
_____ 14. Hydrocephalus
_____ 15. Degenerative arthritis
_____ 16. Pleural effusion
_____ 17. Osteoma
_____ 18. Bowel obstruction
_____ 19. Osteopetrosis
_____ 20. Fibrosarcoma
_____ 21. Acites
_____ 22. Neuroblastoma
_____ 23. Cirrhosis of liver
_____ 24. Metastasis
_____ 25. Bronchiectasis

Answer Key	Notes
1. A	
2. B	
3. A	
4. B	
5. A	
6. A	
7. B	
8. A	
9. B	
10. A	
11. B	
12. A	
13. B	
14. A	
15. B	
16. A	
17. A	
18. B	
19. A	
20. B	
21. A	
22. B	
23. A	
24. B	
25. A	

Exercise 3-7 Image Production and Evaluation

DIRECTIONS: Use each answer only once.

A. Synergism
B. Exposure latitude
C. Blotchiness
D. Estar
E. Sensitometric
F. Kilovoltage
G. Grid cutoff
H. Motion
I. Resolution
J. Involuntary
K. Quantum mottle
L. Intensification factor
M. Afterglow
N. Reciprocity law
O. Protective
P. Fog
Q. Cesium iodide
R. Foreshortening and elongation
S. True distortion
T. Luminescence
U. Antistatic
V. Archiving
W. Parallel
X. Mach effect
Y. Lanthanum

_____ 1. Process of preparing a film for long-term storage
_____ 2. Nonuniform distribution of densities of graininess
_____ 3. Continuous emission of light after phosphor stimulation
_____ 4. Density of film is proportional to exposure intensity × duration
_____ 5. Shape distortion is also known as
_____ 6. Poor alignment of the anatomical part, film, and tube results in
_____ 7. Sum of two agents working together is greater than the agents working alone
_____ 8. Shiny/dull area on film from uneven drying
_____ 9. Layer of intensifying screen closest to the film
_____ 10. Range between minimum and maximum exposure density
_____ 11. Base used in subtraction film
_____ 12 Undesirable absorption of primary radiation
_____ 13. Ideal type of grid for portables and/or stretcher cases
_____ 14. Motion attributed to physiological action
_____ 15. Single most detrimental factor of unsharpness
_____ 16. Special screen cleansers contain compounds that are
_____ 17. Curve used for sensitivity, latitude, density, and contrast
_____ 18. Varies with thickness of the part by 2/centimeter
_____ 19. Most significant factor in loss of image visibility
_____ 20. Ratio of exposure compared with and without screens
_____ 21. Rare earth phosphor compound
_____ 22. Number of line pairs/mm recorded
_____ 23. Occurs when the eye perceives a boundary
_____ 24. Component of a fluoroscopic screen
_____ 25. Ability of a material to emit light

Answer Key	Notes
1. V	
2. K	
3. M	
4. N	
5. S	
6. R	
7. A	
8. C	
9. O	
10. B	
11. D	
12. G	
13. W	
14. J	
15. H	
16. U	
17. E	
18. F	
19. P	
20. L	
21. Y	
22. I	
23. X	
24. Q	
25. T	

Exercise 3-8 mA, Time, and mAs Problems

A. 40 mAs	G. 120 mAs	M. 1/4 sec	S. 250 mA
B. 60 mAs	H. 30 mAs	N. 1 sec	T. 50 mA
C. 90 mAs	I. 4/5 sec	O. 1/20 sec	U. 100 mA
D. 100 mAs	J. 1/5 sec	P. 800 mA	V. 25 mA
E. 150 mAs	K. 1/2 sec	Q. 1200 mA	W. 300 mA
F. 300 mAs	L. 1/120 sec	R. 75 mA	X. 200 mA

DIRECTIONS: In items 1 to 8, assign the correct mAs quantity. Use choices A–H. Use each answer only once.

_____ 1. 100 mA at 6/10 sec = _____mAs
_____ 2. 200 mA at 1 1/2 sec = _____mAs
_____ 3. 400 mA at 1/4 sec = _____mAs
_____ 4. 300 mA at 1/2 sec = _____mAs
_____ 5. 100 mA at 2/5 sec = _____mAs
_____ 6. 200 mA at 3/5 sec = _____mAs
_____ 7. 300 mA at 3/10 sec = _____mAs
_____ 8. 50 mA at 3/5 sec = _____mAs

DIRECTIONS: In items 9 to 15, assign the correct time quantity. Use choices I–O. Use each answer only once.

_____ 9. 200 mA 1/2 sec = 400 mA _____sec
_____ 10. 100 mA 1/10 sec = 200 mA _____sec
_____ 11. 300 mA 1/5 sec = 75 mA _____sec
_____ 12. 100 mA 1/30 sec = 400 mA _____sec
_____ 13. 50 mA 2 sec = 200 mA _____sec
_____ 14. 400 mA 1/20 sec = 100 mA _____sec
_____ 15. 200 mA 1/4 sec = 50 mA _____sec

DIRECTIONS: In items 16 to 24, assign the correct mA quantity. Use choices P–X. Use each answer only once.

_____ 16. 100 mA 1/8 sec = _____mA 1/2 sec
_____ 17. 200 mA 1/20 sec = _____mA 1/80 sec
_____ 18. 400 mA 1/5 sec = _____mA 4/5 sec
_____ 19. 300 mA 1/10 sec = _____mA 1/40 sec
_____ 20. 150 mA 1/40 sec = _____mA 1/20 sec
_____ 21. 100 mA 1/2 sec = _____mA 1/5 sec
_____ 22. 200 mA 1/30 sec = _____mA 1/8 sec
_____ 23. 400 mA 1/20 sec = _____mA 1/15 sec
_____ 24. 50 mA 3/5 sec = _____mA 3/20 sec

Answer Key	Notes
1. B	
2. F	
3. D	
4. E	
5. A	
6. G	
7. C	
8. H	
9. M	
10. O	
11. I	
12. L	
13. K	
14. J	
15. N	
16. V	
17. P	
18. U	
19. Q	
20. R	
21. S	
22. T	
23. W	
24. X	

Exercise 3-9 mA, Time, kV and Screens

A. Slow (detail) (50)
B. Par (medium) (100)
C. High (200)
D. Rare earth (400)
E. 60 kV
F. 150 mA
G. 65 kV
H. 3/10 sec
I. 55 kV
J. 100 mA
K. 75 kV
L. 80 kV
M. 1/10 sec
N. 1/15 sec
O. 3/5 sec
P. 92 kV
Q. 225 mA
R. 1/4 sec
S. 25 mA

DIRECTIONS: In items 1 to 8, match the type of screen to each item. Use choices A–D. Answers may be used more than once.

_____	1.	200	1/2	70	par	=	400	1/4	80	_____
_____	2.	300	1/20	70	slow	=	150	1/40	60	_____
_____	3.	500	1/10	60	high	=	250	1/5	70	_____
_____	4.	100	1/4	80	slow	=	200	1/16	92	_____
_____	5.	200	1/4	60	rare earth	=	100	1/2	70	_____
_____	6.	400	1/16	70	par	=	100	1/8	60	_____
_____	7.	50	1/2	56	par	=	100	1/4	65	_____
_____	8.	400	1/10	92	high	=	200	2/5	104	_____

DIRECTIONS: In items 9 to 23, assign the correct voltage, amperage, or time to each item. Use choices E–S. Use each answer only once.

_____	9.	200	1/4	70	par	=	100	1/8	_____	high
_____	10.	100	1/2	55	par	=	50	2	_____	slow
_____	11.	300	3/10	80	par	=	150	_____	92	slow
_____	12.	50	4/5	65	high	=	200	2/5	_____	slow
_____	13.	400	1/20	60	High	=	100	_____	70	high
_____	14.	200	1/4	60	par	=	100	1/8	_____	rare earth
_____	15.	25	1/10	75	par	=	100	1/40	_____	high
_____	16.	100	3/10	70	par	=	100	3/20	_____	slow
_____	17.	400	3/20	60	par	=	100	_____	70	par
_____	18.	200	1/2	65	high	=	_____	1	75	rare earth
_____	19.	300	3/20	70	par	=	_____	3/5	55	par
_____	20.	100	1/10	75	par	=	_____	1/20	80	par
_____	21.	100	1/4	80	par	=	_____	1/16	92	high
_____	22.	200	1/60	70	high	=	100	_____	80	slow
_____	23.	400	1/16	60	par	=	200	_____	50	par

Answer Key	Notes
1. A	
2. D	
3. B	
4. A	
5. C	
6. D	
7. A	
8. A	
9. L	
10. I	
11. O	
12. K	
13. M	
14. E	
15. G	
16. P	
17. H	
18. S	
19. Q	
20. F	
21. J	
22. N	
23. R	

Exercise 3-10 Grid Conversions, mAs, Distance, and Inverse Square Law

A. 8:1 grid
B. 120 mAs
C. 400 mAs
D. 72 mAs
E. 60 mAs
F. 1 sec
G. 92 kV
H. ⅓ sec
I. 150 mAs
J. 97.6 mAs
K. 27 mAs
L. 135 mAs
M. 50in. FFD
N. 15 mAs
O. 1/20 sec
P. 28.8 mAs
Q. 256 mAs
R. 0.9 sec
S. 300 mAs
T. 45 mR
U. 194.4 mAs
V. ⅕ sec
W. 48 mR

DIRECTIONS: In items 1 to 10, assign the proper answer. Use choices A–I. Answers may be used more than once.

_____ 1. No grid 50 mAs = 6:1 grid _____mAs
_____ 2. No grid 80 mAs = 10:1 grid _____mAs
_____ 3. No grid 200 mA ⅕ sec = 12:1 grid 200 MA _____sec
_____ 4. No grid 300 mA 1/20 sec = _____grid 300 mA ⅕ sec
_____ 5. 5:1 grid 75 mAs = 8:1 grid _____mAs
_____ 6. 10:1 grid 120 mAs = 6:1 grid _____mAs
_____ 7. 8:1 grid 150 mA ½ = 12:1 grid 300 mA _____sec
_____ 8. No grid 80 mAs 75 kV = 6:1 grid _____mAs 86 kV
_____ 9. 8:1 grid 120 mAs 80 kV = 5:1 grid 30 mAs _____kV
_____ 10. 12:1 grid 100 mAs 90 kV = 6:1 _____mAs 90 kV

DIRECTIONS: In items 11 to 24, assign the correct quantity. Use choices J–W. Use each answer only once.

_____ 11. 60 mAs at 72in. = _____mAs at 36in.
_____ 12. 60 mAs at 40in. = _____mAs at 60in.
_____ 13. 400 mAs at 50in. = _____mAs at 40in.
_____ 14. 250 mAs at 40in. = _____mAs at 25in.
_____ 15. 675 mAs at 63in. = _____mAs at 42in.
_____ 16. 80 mAs at 40in. = _____mAs at 24in
_____ 17. 70 mAs at 36in. = _____mAs at 60in.
_____ 18. 75 mAs at 25in. = 300 mAs at_____in.
_____ 19. 300 mA at ¼ sec and 50in. = _____mAs at 30
_____ 20. 50 mA at ⅗ sec and 72in. = 50mA at_____sec and 36in.
_____ 21. 700 mA at 3/10 and 80in. = 700 mA at_____sec and 40in.
_____ 22. 300 mA at ⅕ and 42in. = 150 mA at_____sec and 63in.
_____ 23. 12 mR at 72in. FFD = _____mR at 36in. (dosage)
_____ 24. 20 mR at 72in. FFD = _____mR at 48in. (dose)

Answer Key	Notes
1. I	
2. C	
3. F	
4. A	
5. I	
6. D	
7. H	
8. B	
9. G	
10. E	
11. N	
12. L	
13. Q	
14. J	
15. S	
16. P	
17. U	
18. M	
19. K	
20. V	
21. O	
22. R	
23. W	
24. T	

Exercise 3-11 Problems and Calculations

DIRECTIONS: Calculate the missing factor. Use each answer only once.

A. 92 kV
B. 200 mAs
C. 2.5 ohms
D. 76 kV
E. 50 mAs
F. 84 kV
G. 72 degrees
H. 150 mA
I. 56 kV
J. 120 mAs
K. 0.2 sec
L. 106 kV
M. 100 mA
N. 100 V
O. 64 degrees
P. 7000
Q. 75 mAs
R. 60 kV
S. 300 mA
T. 25 mAs
U. 225 mAs
V. 80 kV
W. 1 sec
X. 166 mAs
Y. 400 mAs

_____ 1. 300 ¼ 60 par = _____⅛ 70 high
_____ 2. 200 ½ 80 passing 1 HVL = _____½ 80 kV
_____ 3. 300 mA 8:1 grid = _____mAs at TT
_____ 4. 100 ⅕ 70 par = 200 ⅒ _____high
_____ 5. 50 A and 2 ohms = _____V
_____ 6. 100 mAs at 6:1 grid = _____mAs (maintained) for 12:1 grid
_____ 7. 100 mAs needed at 40in. _____mAs at 60in. (required)
_____ 8. 150 mAs at 16:1 grid = _____mAs to TT
_____ 9. 200 mA ½ sec × 70 kV = _____HU
_____ 10. 3 min at 68 degrees developer = 4 min at _____degrees
_____ 11. 100 mA ½ sec 80 kV = 50 mA ¼ sec _____kV (same density)
_____ 12. 200 mAs at 80 kV = 100 mAs at _____kV
_____ 13. 100 mAs at 60 kV to double density = _____mAs
_____ 14. 100 mAs TT to 8:1 grid = _____mAs
_____ 15. 60 mAs 6:1 grid = _____mAs at 16:1 grid
_____ 16. 100 ½ 74 for 20 cm = 100 ½ _____kV for 25 cm
_____ 17. 100 1/20 cassette = 100 _____CBH
_____ 18. 5 min at 68 degrees developer = 4 min at _____degrees
_____ 19. 200 ½ 70 = 100 ½_____to increase scale of contrast but hold density
_____ 20. 400 mAs passing through 3 HVLs=_____mAs
_____ 21. 300 mA at 60 mAs = (time)_____
_____ 22. 200 1/30 70–20 cm chest measures 23 = _____kV
_____ 23. 100 V and 4 A = _____ohms
_____ 24. 300 mA ½ sec 70 kV par = _____mA ¼ sec 70 kV high
_____ 25. 100 1/30 52 kV for 3 cm = 100 1/30 _____kV for 5 cm

Answer Key	Notes
1. H	
2. M	
3. Q	
4. R	
5. N	
6. X	
7. U	
8. T	
9. P	
10. O	
11. L	
12. A	
13. B	
14. Y	
15. J	
16. F	
17. W	
18. G	
19. V	
20. E	
21. K	
22. D	
23. C	
24. S	
25. I	

Exercise 3-12 Radiographic Technique

DIRECTIONS: Use each answer only once.

A. Inverse square law
B. 80 kV
C. 15% rule
D. 20 to 25 kV
E. 2 kV
F. 20 mAs
G. 2 × mAs
H. 30%
I. Quantity
J. 16:1
K. 2 × mAs + 10% kV
L. kVp
M. 100 to 120 kV
N. ¼ of original
O. ½ exposure time
P. 40in.
Q. 48 to 52 kV
R. +12 cm or above 60 kV
S. 2.5 mm
T. Quality
U. Caliper
V. Low kV
W. mAs
X. AEC
Y. 500 milliseconds

_____ 1. Device used to measure patient thickness
_____ 2. Related to kV employed
_____ 3. Guideline for using Bucky
_____ 4. Requires to penetrate barium
_____ 5. Standard SID for table procedures
_____ 6. Needed to maintain density when doubling mA
_____ 7. Utilized in soft-tissue demonstration
_____ 8. Controls radiographic density
_____ 9. Adjustment for +1 cm
_____ 10. Required aluminum filtration
_____ 11. Formula relating to dosage and distance
_____ 12. Phototimed units are referred to as _____
_____ 13. Minimum mAs change to show density
_____ 14. Equivalent to 200 mA at ⅒ sec
_____ 15. Intensity produced when SID is doubled
_____ 16. Factor that controls level of contrast
_____ 17. Equivalent to 2 × mAs
_____ 18. Equivalent to ½ or 0.5 sec
_____ 19. Proper adjustment for cast
_____ 20. Recommended kV level for urographic study
_____ 21. Adjustment needed to go from 14 × 17 field to 8 × 10 field
_____ 22. Penetration required for a 3-cm object
_____ 23. Grid required for high-kV studies
_____ 24. kV used to radiograph specimens
_____ 25. Related to mAs employed

Answer Key	Notes
1. U	
2. T	
3. R	
4. M	
5. P	
6. O	
7. V	
8. W	
9. E	
10. S	
11. A	
12. X	
13. H	
14. F	
15. N	
16. L	
17. C	
18. Y	
19. K	
20. B	
21. G	
22. Q	
23. J	
24. D	
25. I	

Exercise 3-13 X-Ray Film and Intensifying Screens

DIRECTIONS: Use each answer only once.

A. Calcium tungstate
B. Negative
C. Cellulose acetate
D. Lag
E. Latent
F. Gelatin
G. Radiolucent
H. Gadolinium
I. Duplitized
J. Characteristic
K. Radiopaque
L. 5%
M. AgBr (halide)
N. Barium lead sulfate
O. Total density
P. Nonscreen film
Q. Orthochromatic
R. Manifest
S. Photographic effect
T. Supercoating
U. 95%
V. Remnant
W. Latitude
X. Processing
Y. Polyester

_____ 1. Invisible image produced
_____ 2. High-speed screen composition
_____ 3. Density from x-ray when using screens
_____ 4. Absorbs x-ray beam
_____ 5. Percent of image recorded from screens
_____ 6. Transforms latent to manifest
_____ 7. Processed image
_____ 8. Protects emulsion from scratching
_____ 9. X-ray film base used 20 to 25 years ago
_____ 10. Medium and slow-speed screen composition
_____ 11. Requires 100% x-ray
_____ 12. Modern x-ray film base
_____ 13. X-rays that form image
_____ 14. Film coated on both sides
_____ 15. Rare earth phosphor
_____ 16. Finished radiograph
_____ 17. Colloid that allows chemicals to act
_____ 18. Curve that plots radiographic densities
_____ 19. Recording of images in ranges of tones
_____ 20. Green-sensitive film
_____ 21. X-ray film emulsion
_____ 22. After glow of screens
_____ 23. Film completely black
_____ 24. Easily penetrated
_____ 25. Formation of the latent image

Answer Key	Notes
1. E	
2. N	
3. L	
4. K	
5. U	
6. X	
7. R	
8. T	
9. C	
10. A	
11. P	
12. Y	
13. V	
14. I	
15. H	
16. B	
17. F	
18. J	
19. W	
*20. Q	
21. M	
22. D	
23. O	
24. G	
25. S	

Exercise 3-14 Film Processing

DIRECTIONS: Use each answer only once.

A. Replenishment rate
B. Microswitch
C. Pi lines
D. Transport rollers
E. Chemical fog
F. Crossover rack
G. Negative
H. Transport system
I. Phenidone
J. Turnaround assembly
K. GBX-2 filter
L. Emulsion pick-off
M. Master roller
N. static artifact
O. dichroic
P. Replenishment system
Q. Aldehydes
R. Sensitive speck
S. Guide shoes
T. Manual processing
U. Hypo
V. Temperature control system
W. Wetting agent
X. Rinsing
Y. Fixer neutralizer

_____ 1. Caused by dirty or warped rollers
_____ 2. Rapid processing developer agent
_____ 3. Maintain 95°F by a heating element
_____ 4. Occurs for 30 sec between developer and fixer
_____ 5. Curved metal lip to direct film around bend
_____ 6. Best results at temperatures of 68 to 72°F
_____ 7. Meters into each tank proper amounts of solution
_____ 8. Crown, tree, and smudge
_____ 9. Term used for all chemical stains
_____ 10. Solar roller with plastic guide shoes
_____ 11. Fixing agents are known as
_____ 12. Acts as development center for entire crystal
_____ 13. Smaller rack composed of rollers and guide shoes
_____ 14. Antifogging agents for high temperatures
_____ 15. Reduces drying time by 50%
_____ 16. Set so 60 to 70 mL of developer per 14in. of film
_____ 17. Uniform dull gray
_____ 18. Rollers, transport racks, and drive motor
_____ 19. Artifact occurring at 3.1416-in. intervals
_____ 20. Located at bottom of transport rack assembly
_____ 21. Conveys film along its path
_____ 22. Finished radiograph
_____ 23. Controls replenishment rate of chemicals
_____ 24. Added to reduce washing time
_____ 25. Used over 15-W bulb in darkroom

Answer Key	Notes
1. L	
2. I	
3. V	
4. X	
5. S	
6. T	
7. P	
8. N	
9. O	
10. M	
11. U	
12. R	
13. F	
14. Q	
15. W	
16. A	
17. E	
18. H	
19. C	
20. J	
21. D	
22. G	
23. B	
24. Y	
25. K	

Exercise 3-15 Darkroom Solutions

DIRECTIONS: Use each answer only once.

A. Potassium bromide
B. Below 60°F
C. Hydroquinone
D. 28% acetic acid
E. Sodium sulfite
F. Contamination
G. Phenidone
H. Potassium alum
I. Glutaraledehyde
J. Water
K. Detergent
L. 5 min at 68°F
M. Ammonium thiosulfate
N. Temperature above 75°F
O. 3 gal/min
P. Permanence of image
Q. 95°F
R. Aerial oxidation
S. Elon
T. Sodium carbonate
U. 2 × developer
V. 6BX
W. Acetic acid
X. Milkiness
Y. 3 months

_____ 1. Neutralizes the developer (activator)
_____ 2. Shortens hand tank's solution life
_____ 3. Produces shades of gray rapidly
_____ 4. Archival quality
_____ 5. Removes undeveloped AgBr (clearing agent)
_____ 6. Wetting agent
_____ 7. Antifog agent (restrainer)
_____ 8. Filter used in darkroom
_____ 9. Produces black tones slowly
_____ 10. Normal developer temperature (i.e., automatic processor
_____ 11. Air introduced to chemical when mixing
_____ 12. Underexposed or developed AgBr
_____ 13. Controls oxidation (preservative)
_____ 14. Used in developer to build up detail
_____ 15. Helps swell gelatin (activator)
_____ 16. Fixer in developer
_____ 17. Optimum time and temperature
_____ 18. Shrinks and stiffens emulsion (hardener)
_____ 19. Automatic processor hardener
_____ 20. Exhaustion limit for hand tanks
_____ 21. Dissolves chemicals for use (solvent)
_____ 22. Hydroquinone will not function
_____ 23. Stopbath component
_____ 24. Minimum flow rate for processor's wash tank
_____ 25. Time film is in fixer

Answer Key

Notes

1. W
2. N
3. G
4. P
5. M
6. K
7. A
8. V
9. C
10. Q
11. R
12. X
13. E
14. S
15. T
16. F
17. L
18. H
19. I
20. Y
21. J
22. B
23. D
24. O
25. U

Exercise 3-16 Darkroom and Film Artifacts

DIRECTIONS: Use each answer only once.

A. Crescents
B. Mottled
C. Pi lines
D. Bleached
E. Patterned lines
F. Static
G. Reticulation
H. Fuzzy image
I. Reverse image
J. Overexposure
K. Crinkle, half-moon
L. Fog
M. Opalescent
N. Air bubbles
O. White specks
P. Blank film
Q. Aerial oxidation
R. Sticky
S. Guide marks
T. Incorrect density
U. Light leak
V. Streaks, greasy
W. Exposed band
X. Scratched film
Y. Dirty film

_____ 1. Regularly spaced scratches
_____ 2. Bending of film
_____ 3. Grooves on film from rollers
_____ 4. No x-ray exposure
_____ 5. Blistering from different temperature
_____ 6. Excessive density around film edge
_____ 7. Uniform spots
_____ 8. Shiny film from fresh fixer
_____ 9. Improper mAs/kVp values
_____ 10. Oxidized solutions with air
_____ 11. Poor film–screen contact
_____ 12. Old film
_____ 13. Hair, dust, or barium in/on cassette
_____ 14. Over- or underreplenishment
_____ 15. Left in fixer too long
_____ 16. Clogged filter
_____ 17. Film stacked improperly
_____ 18. Film exposed in box
_____ 19. Turn on light with film in developer
_____ 20. kVp value too high
_____ 21. Branch- or treelike mark
_____ 22. Film not completely washed
_____ 23. Dryer thermostat too low
_____ 24. Images from grid
_____ 25. Improperly seated rollers

Answer Key	Notes
1. S	
2. K	
3. C	
4. P	
5. G	
6. U	
7. N	
8. M	
9. J	
10. Q	
11. H	
12. B	
13. O	
14. T	
15. D	
16. Y	
17. A	
18. W	
19. I	
20. L	
21. F	
22. V	
23. R	
24. E	
25. X	

Exercise 3-17 Grids

DIRECTIONS: Use each answer only once.

A. High-kV technique
B. 16:1
C. Fog
D. Crosshatch
E. Aluminum or plastic fiber
F. 2 to 3 cm
G. Grid lines
H. Cleanup
I. Rhombic
J. Bucky
K. Ratio
L. 75%
M. Selectivity
N. Lead
O. Grid cutoff
P. Contrast
Q. Patient size above 12 cm
R. Moving grid
S. 3:1 and 6:1 moving grid
T. Interspace
U. Air gap
V. Radii
W. 8:1 grid
X. Scatter radiation
Y. Patient dose

_____ 1. Undesirable absorption of the primary beam
_____ 2. Increase OFD to absorb scatter radiation
_____ 3. Only real disadvantage in using a grid
_____ 4. Decreases radiographic contrast
_____ 5. Distance from tube to grid
_____ 6. Approximate cleanup of a 5:1 grid
_____ 7. Requires use of a grid
_____ 8. Interspace materials for most grids
_____ 9. Needs the use of a grid with a high ratio
_____ 10. Lead strips running parallel to long and short axes
_____ 11. Sections of radiolucent materials
_____ 12. Grid utilized in mammography
_____ 13. Good cleanup with lead strips at right angles
_____ 14. Occurs with high incident of scatter
_____ 15. Requires four times more mAs than TT technique
_____ 16. Potter–Bucky diaphragm (recipromatic)
_____ 17. Ability to remove a high percentage of scatter
_____ 18. Ratio of transmitted primary radiation to transmitted scatter
_____ 19. Strips found in grid
_____ 20. Utilized for high-kVp mAs exposures
_____ 21. Degree of difference between the light and dark areas of the film
_____ 22. Images when primary beam absorbed by grid
_____ 23. Height of lead strips to distance between them
_____ 24. Distance single-stroke grid moves
_____ 25. Inventor of the grid in 1913

Answer Key	Notes
1. O	
2. U	
3. Y	
4. X	
5. V	
6. L	
7. Q	
8. E	
9. A	
10. D	
11. T	
12. S	
13. I	
14. C	
15. W	
16. R	
17. H	
18. M	
19. N	
20. B	
21. P	
22. G	
23. K	
24. F	
25. J	

Section 4
Radiographic Procedures

Exercise 4-1 Anatomical and Positioning Terms

DIRECTIONS: Use each answer only once.

A. Inferior
B. Medial
C. Distal
D. Frontal or coronal plane
E. Posterior
F. Supine
G. Anterior
H. Invert
I. Transverse plane
J. Visceral
K. Flex
L. Internal
M. Sagittal plane
N. Plantar
O. Prone
P. Midsagittal plane
Q. Abduct
R. Superior
S. Lateral
T. Rotate
U. Proximal
V. Longitudinal
W. Cephalic
X. Evert
Y. Extend

_____ 1. On the inside of the body
_____ 2. Makes superior and inferior segments
_____ 3. Refers to the head
_____ 4. Makes right and left segments
_____ 5. To straighten or stretch out
_____ 6. Upper part of body
_____ 7. Relating to an organ itself
_____ 8. Makes equal right and left parts
_____ 9. Part of structure closest to source
_____ 10. Away from the midline
_____ 11. To bend
_____ 12. Makes anterior and posterior segments
_____ 13. To turn outward
_____ 14. Back portion of the body
_____ 15. Part located nearest median line
_____ 16. Lengthwise or along the long axis
_____ 17. Lying on back (AP)
_____ 18. To turn along one axis
_____ 19. Part farthest away from source
_____ 20. Refers to the lower part
_____ 21. Lying face down (PA)
_____ 22. Front portion of the body
_____ 23. To turn inward
_____ 24. Draw away from midline
_____ 25. Refers to sole of the foot

Answer Key	Notes
1. L	
2. I	
3. W	
4. M	
5. Y	
6. R	
7. J	
8. P	
9. U	
10. S	
11. K	
12. D	
13. X	
14. E	
15. B	
16. V	
17. F	
18. T	
19. C	
20. A	
21. O	
22. G	
23. H	
24. Q	
25. N	

Exercise **4-2**

Anatomic Lines, Planes, and Regions

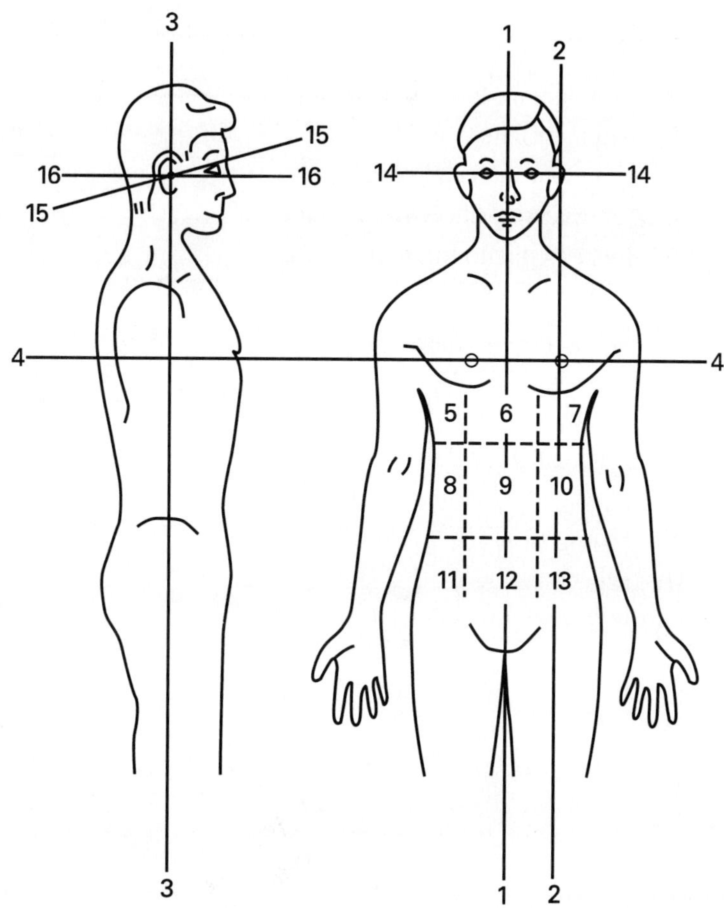

Plate 5 (Artwork courtesy of William F. Toeppe)

Plate 5. Anatomic Lines, Planes, and Regions

Identify the structures labeled 1 to 16.

1.	9.
2.	10.
3.	11.
4.	12.
5.	13.
6.	14.
7.	15.
8.	16.

Plate 5. Anatomic Lines, Planes, and Regions

1. Midsagittal plane (median line)
2. Sagittal plane
3. Frontal or coronal plane
4. Transverse or horizontal plane
5. Right hypochondriac region
6. Epigastric region
7. Left hypochondriac region
8. Right lumbar region
9. Umbilical region
10. Left lumbar region
11. Right iliac (inguinal) region
12. Hypogastric (pubic) region
13. Left iliac (inguinal) region
14. Interorbital or interpupillary line
15. Orbitomeatal or canthomeatal line
16. Infraorbitomeatal (Reid's) baseline

Exercise 4-3 Body Regions and Quadrants

A. Right upper quadrant
B. Right lower quadrant
C. Left upper quadrant
D. Left lower quadrant
E. Right hypochondriac
F. Epigastric
G. Left hypochondriac
H. Right lumbar
I. Umbilical
J. Left lumbar
K. Right iliac
L. Hypogastric
M. Left iliac

DIRECTIONS: In Items 1 to 14, identify the relevant quadrant for each anatomical structure. Use choices A–D. Answers may be used more than once.

_____ 1. Gallbladder
_____ 2. Terminal ileum
_____ 3. Left middle ureter (middle of left ureter)
_____ 4. Duodenum
_____ 5. Left kidney
_____ 6. Head of pancreas
_____ 7. Appendix
_____ 8. Spleen
_____ 9. Greater part of liver
_____ 10. Lower descending colon
_____ 11. Lower ascending colon
_____ 12. Cecum (usually)
_____ 13. Bile Ducts
_____ 14. Upper descending colon

DIRECTIONS: In items 15 to 24, identify the relevant region for each anatomical structure. Use choices E–M. Answers may be used more than once.

_____ 15. Cecum
_____ 16. Greater curvature of stomach
_____ 17. Jejunum
_____ 18. Flexure of sigmoid colon
_____ 19. Ileocecal valve
_____ 20. Appendix
_____ 21. Hepatic flexure of colon
_____ 22. Most of transverse colon
_____ 23. Ascending colon
_____ 24. Gallbladder

Answer Key

Notes

1. A
2. B
3. D
4. A
5. C
6. A
7. B
8. C
9. A
10. D
11. B
12. B
13. A
14. C
15. K
16. G
17. M
18. L
19. K
20. K
21. E
22. I
23. H
24. F

Exercise 4-4 Vertebral Levels

DIRECTIONS: Answers may be used more than once.

A. C3
B. T11
C. T4–T5
D. T10
E. C7
F. C5–C6
G. L4–L5
H. T8
I. L5–S1
J. T5
K. L2
L. C4
M. L3
N. D12–L2
O. T9
P. C1
Q. T–12
R. S–2
S. T2–T3

_____ 1. Kidneys
_____ 2. Atlantooccipital articulation
_____ 3. Mastoid process
_____ 4. Clavicles (medial articulation)
_____ 5. Suprasternal (jugular) notch
_____ 6. Umbilicus
_____ 7. Iliac crest
_____ 8. Sternal angle
_____ 9. Angle of mandible (gonion)
_____ 10. Trachea bifurcation
_____ 11. Thyroid cartilage
_____ 12. Nipple
_____ 13. Dome of diaphragm
_____ 14. Vertebra prominens
_____ 15. Gallbladder
_____ 16. Lumbosacral articulation
_____ 17. Lower costal margin
_____ 18. Cricoid cartilage
_____ 19. Anterior superior iliac spine (A.S.I.S.)
_____ 20. Xiphisternal joint
_____ 21. Hyoid bone
_____ 22. Bifurcation to right and left common iliacs
_____ 23. Spinal cord intact ends
_____ 24. Esophagus ends and connects to stomach
_____ 25. Last set of ribs attached

Answer Key

Notes

1. N
2. P
3. P
4. C
5. S
6. M
7. G
8. C
9. A
10. J
11. F
12. H
13. D
14. E
15. N
16. I
17. M
18. F
19. R
20. O
21. L
22. G
23. K
24. B
25. Q

Exercise 4-5 Basic Terminology: Prefix and Suffix

DIRECTIONS: Use each answer only once.

A. Ento
B. Bi or bis
C. Macro
D. Anti, Contra
E. Hemi
F. Poly
G. Hydro
H. Infra
I. Trans
J. Peri
K. Epi
L. Oma
M. Extra
N. Dys
O. Ptosis
P. Ecto
Q. Otomy
R. Retro
S. Less
T. Post
U. Ostomy
V. Inter
W. itis
X. Algia
Y. Lith

_____ 1. Refers to water
_____ 2. After
_____ 3. Below
_____ 4. Outside or beyond
_____ 5. Behind
_____ 6. Pain
_____ 7. Difficult
_____ 8. Outer
_____ 9. Against
_____ 10. Among or between
_____ 11. Half
_____ 12. Inside
_____ 13. Upon
_____ 14. Mouth or opening
_____ 15. Two or twice
_____ 16. Stone
_____ 17. Across
_____ 18. Around
_____ 19. Inflammation
_____ 20. Falling down
_____ 21. Too much or many
_____ 22. Tumor
_____ 23. Large
_____ 24. Without
_____ 25. Incision or cut

Answer Key	Notes
1. G	
2. T	
3. H	
4. M	
5. R	
6. X	
7. N	
8. P	
9. D	
10. V	
11. E	
12. A	
13. K	
14. U	
15. B	
16. Y	
17. I	
18. J	
19. W	
20. O	
21. F	
22. L	
23. C	
24. S	
25. Q	

Exercise 4-6 Medical Terminology

DIRECTIONS: Use each answer only once.

A. Dolicho
B. Brachi
C. Hemo
D. Acou
E. Cranio
F. Ectasis
G. Carcin
H. Cardi
I. Entero
J. Esthesia
K. Adeno
L. Genito
M. Cysto
N. Costa
O. Glosso
P. Chondr
Q. Erythro
R. Brady
S. Glyco
T. Gyn
U. Derma
V. Chole
W. Gram
X. Gastro
Y. Hepato

_____ 1. Skin
_____ 2. Ribs
_____ 3. Arm
_____ 4. Bladder
_____ 5. Heart
_____ 6 Small
_____ 7. Bile, gall
_____ 8. Hearing
_____ 9. Red
_____ 10. Dilatation
_____ 11. Slow
_____ 12. Stomach
_____ 13. Long
_____ 14. Tongue
_____ 15. Gland
_____ 16. Record
_____ 17. Sensation
_____ 18. Skull
_____ 19. Cancer
_____ 20. Blood
_____ 21. Reproduction organs
_____ 22. Liver
_____ 23. Cartilage
_____ 24. Female
_____ 25. Sweet

Answer Key	Notes
1. U	
2. N	
3. B	
4. M	
5. H	
6. I	
7. V	
8. D	
9. Q	
10. F	
11. R	
12. X	
13. A	
14. O	
15. K	
16. W	
17. J	
18. E	
19. G	
20. C	
21. L	
22. Y	
23. P	
24. T	
25. S	

Exercise 4-7 Medical Terminology

DIRECTIONS: Use each answer only once.

A. Aphasia
B. Sclero
C. Psycho
D. Achondroplasia
E. Reno
F. Viscero
G. Steno
H. Pulmono
I. Aneurysm
J. Scolio
K. Aphagia
L. Salpingo
M. Anomaly
N. Abscess
O. Asceptic
P. Pyo
Q. Adipose
R. Thermo
S. Atrophic
T. Septic
U. Ataxia
V. Ascites
W. Angioma
X. Bifurcate
Y. Atresia

_____ 1. Abnormality
_____ 2. Tube
_____ 3. Fat
_____ 4. Mind
_____ 5. Area of tissue breakdown
_____ 6. Poison
_____ 7. Tumor made of blood vessels
_____ 8. Kidney
_____ 9. Accumulation of abdominal fluid
_____ 10. Pus
_____ 11. Weakening of vessel wall
_____ 12. Narrowed
_____ 13. Hardness
_____ 14. Free of infection
_____ 15. Heat
_____ 16. Large head and short extremities
_____ 17. Lung
_____ 18. Wasting away
_____ 19. Internal organs
_____ 20. Not eating
_____ 21. Twisted
_____ 22. Divide in two
_____ 23. Abnormal closure of a passage
_____ 24. Loss of speech
_____ 25. Lack of muscular coordination

Answer Key	Notes
1. M	
2. L	
3. Q	
4. C	
5. N	
6. T	
7. W	
8. E	
9. V	
10. P	
11. I	
12. G	
13. B	
14. O	
15. R	
16. D	
17. H	
18. S	
19. F	
20. K	
21. J	
22. X	
23. Y	
24. A	
25. U	

Exercise 4-8 Terminology: Prefix and Suffix

DIRECTIONS: Use each answer only once.

A. Malacia
B. Pathy
C. Osteo
D. Carcin
E. Odont
F. Leuko
G. Neuro
H. Oculo
I. Hyster
J. Ovo
K. Penia
L. Masto
M. Phago
N. Idio
O. Phlebo
P. Neo
Q. Oma
R. Necro
S. Oophor
T. Mega
U. Pnea
V. Plasty
W. Procto
X. Pod
Y. Phobia

_____ 1. Ovum, egg
_____ 2. Self
_____ 3. Vein
_____ 4. White
_____ 5. Rectum
_____ 6. Foot
_____ 7. Cancer
_____ 8. New
_____ 9. Softening
_____ 10. Bone
_____ 11. To eat
_____ 12. Death
_____ 13. Air
_____ 14. Tumor
_____ 15. Uterus
_____ 16. Molding (repair)
_____ 17. Eye
_____ 18. Teeth
_____ 19. Breast
_____ 20. Lack of
_____ 21. Fear
_____ 22. Nerve
_____ 23. Ovary
_____ 24. Large
_____ 25. Disease

Answer Key	Notes
1. J	
2. N	
3. O	
4. F	
5. W	
6. X	
7. D	
8. P	
9. A	
10. C	
11. M	
12. R	
13. U	
14. Q	
15. I	
16. V	
17. H	
18. E	
19. L	
20. K	
21. Y	
22. G	
23. S	
24. T	
25. B	

Exercise 4-9 Medical Terminology

DIRECTIONS: Use each answer only once.

A. Nephroptosis
B. Leukemia
C. Metastasis
D. Lipoma
E. Nephritis
F. Mastitis
G. Myalgia
H. Necrosis
I. Kyphosis
J. Meningitis
K. Lithiasis
L. Oliguria
M. Osteitis
N. Otitis
O. Leukopenia
P. Osteoma
Q. Neuroma
R. Osteomalacia
S. Neuritis
T. Osteomyelitis
U. Nephroma
V. Meningocele
W. Occlusion
X. Peripheral
Y. Nodule

_____ 1. Tumor of the kidney
_____ 2. Protrusion of membranes around brain and spinal cord
_____ 3. Inflammation of bone tissue
_____ 4. Disorder of blood and increased (WBC)
_____ 5. Softening of bones
_____ 6. Tumor of bone
_____ 7. Inflammation of covering of brain and spinal cord
_____ 8. Ear inflammation
_____ 9. Small solid mass
_____ 10. Inflammation of breast tissue
_____ 11. Related to or located at the surface
_____ 12. Inflammation of a nerve
_____ 13. Condition of stone formation
_____ 14. Diminished amount of urine secretion
_____ 15. Inflammation of the kidney
_____ 16. Terminal spreading of disease
_____ 17. Inflammation of bone by pus-producing organism
_____ 18. Hunchback condition of spine
_____ 19. Tissue death
_____ 20. Process of closing
_____ 21. Muscle pain
_____ 22. Tumor made up of nerve fibers and cells
_____ 23. Decrease in WBC count
_____ 24. Downward displacement of the kidney
_____ 25. Fatty tissue tumor

Answer Key	Notes
1. U	
2. V	
3. M	
4. B	
5. R	
6. P	
7. J	
8. N	
9. Y	
10. F	
11. X	
12. S	
13. K	
14. L	
15. E	
16. C	
17. T	
18. I	
19. H	
20. W	
21. G	
22. Q	
23. O	
24. A	
25. D	

Exercise 4-10 Medical Terminology

DIRECTIONS: Use each answer only once.

A. Sclerosis
B. Sarcoma
C. Pleurisy
D. Tachypnea
E. Stricture
F. Uremia
G. Polyp
H. Salpingitis
I. Prognosis
J. Septicemia
K. Syndrome
L. Pneumonia
M. Varices
N. Urea
O. Pyelitis
P. Spasm
Q. Systole
R. Alopecia
S. Subluxation
T. Fibrosis
U. Psoriasis
V. Urticaria
W. Scoliosis
X. Talipes
Y. Bunions

_____ 1. Hives from a reaction
_____ 2. Inflammation of the kidney pelvis
_____ 3. Enlargements from pressure on great toe
_____ 4. Inflammation of the lungs
_____ 5. Loss of hair (baldness)
_____ 6. Involuntary muscle contraction
_____ 7. Forecast of results of a disorder
_____ 8. Heart muscle contraction phase
_____ 9. Inflammation of connective tissues
_____ 10. Inflammation of the membrane of the lung
_____ 11. Congenital clubfoot
_____ 12. Inflammation of fallopian tube
_____ 13. Enlarged veins
_____ 14 Hardening with loss of elasticity
_____ 15. Scaly skin lesions
_____ 16. Protruding growth from a mucous membrane
_____ 17. Abnormal lateral curvature of spine
_____ 18. Accumulation of waste products in the blood
_____ 19. Tumor made of connective tissue
_____ 20. Rapid breathing
_____ 21. Abnormal narrowing
_____ 22. Group of symptoms indicating a certain disorder
_____ 23. Blood poisoning
_____ 24. Nitrogen waste product
_____ 25. Partial or incomplete dislocation

Answer Key

Notes

1. V
2. O
3. Y
4. L
5. R
6. P
7. I
8. Q
9. T
10. C
11. X
12. H
13. M
14. A
15. U
16. G
17. W
18. F
19. B
20. D
21. E
22. K
23. J
24. N
25. S

Exercise 4-11 Medical Terminology

DIRECTIONS: Use each answer only once.

A. Diaphoresis
B. Calculus
C. Convoluted
D. Dysphagia
E. Cirrhosis
F. Bradycardia
G. Dysentery
H. Colostomy
I. Bronchiectasis
J. Empyema
K. Diastole
L. Chondroma
M. Endocarditis
N. Crepitations
O. Encephalitis
P. Cystitis
Q. Emesis
R. Emphysema
S. Carcinoma
T. Dyspnea
U. Effusion
V. Congenital
W. Edema
X. Diploe
Y. Ectopic

_____ 1. Difficulty in breathing
_____ 2. Liver disorder
_____ 3. Relaxation phase of the heart
_____ 4. Inflammation of the urinary bladder
_____ 5. Present at birth
_____ 6. Abnormal accumulation of fluids
_____ 7. Malignant growth of epithelial cells
_____ 8. Disorder of intestine
_____ 9. Coiled or rolled together
_____ 10. Perspiring
_____ 11. Pulse rate of 60 or less per minute
_____ 12. Vomiting
_____ 13. Sound heard when rubbing fractured bones together
_____ 14. Stone
_____ 15. Escape of fluid into a space
_____ 16. New opening of colon
_____ 17. Accumulation of pus in a cavity
_____ 18. Loss of lung elasticity
_____ 19. Inflammation of the heart wall
_____ 20 Spongy bone in the cranium
_____ 21. Improperly placed
_____ 22. Overgrowth of cartilage tissue
_____ 23. Stagnation of air in lungs
_____ 24. Inflammation of the brain
_____ 25. Difficulty in swallowing

Answer Key	Notes
1. T	
2. E	
3. K	
4. P	
5. V	
6. W	
7. S	
8. G	
9. C	
10. A	
11. F	
12. Q	
13. N	
14. B	
15. U	
16. H	
17. J	
18. I	
19. M	
20. X	
21. Y	
22. L	
23. R	
24. O	
25. D	

Exercise 4-12 Medical Terminology

DIRECTIONS: Use each answer only once.

A. Fistula
B. Epigastrium
C. Eupnea
D. Hematoma
E. Epiglottis
F. Glioma
G. Hydrocephalus
H. Gastritis
I. Epiphysis
J. Idiopathic
K. Hyperglycemia
L. Erythema
M. Hematuria
N. Flatus
O. Hepatitis
P. Infarct
Q. Enteritis
R. Intercostal
S. Hypogastrium
T. Hypertrophy
U. Ischemia
V. Fissure
W. Ileus
X. Hydrocele
Y. Fundus

_____ 1. Lack of sufficient blood to a part
_____ 2. Inflammation of the small bowel
_____ 3. Abnormal accumulation of fluid around brain
_____ 4. Part of hollow organ away from entrance
_____ 5. Redness of skin
_____ 6. Located between the ribs
_____ 7. Blood in the urine
_____ 8. Upper middle section of abdomen
_____ 9. Abnormal passage between two organs
_____ 10. Tissue death from lack of circulation
_____ 11. Normal respiration
_____ 12. Excessive enlargement or overgrowth
_____ 13. Gas in stomach or bowel
_____ 14. Tumor or swelling filled with blood
_____ 15. Lidlike structure covering larynx
_____ 16. Small bowel obstruction
_____ 17. Groove or fold
_____ 18. Increase in sugar in the blood
_____ 19. Tumor of brain or spinal cord
_____ 20. Fluid containing sac or tumor
_____ 21. Inflammation of the liver
_____ 22 End of a long bone
_____ 23. Disorder of unknown origin
_____ 24. Inflammation of the stomach
_____ 25. Lower central region of abdomen

Answer Key

Notes

1. U
2. Q
3. G
4. Y
5. L
6. R
7. M
8. B
9. A
10. P
11. C
12. T
13. N
14. D
15. E
16. W
17. V
18. K
19. F
20. X
21. O
22. I
23. J
24. H
25. S

Exercise 4-13 Anatomical Terms and Conditions

DIRECTIONS: Use each answer only once.

A. Silicosis
B. Septal defect
C. Papilloma
D. Viscosity
E. Achondroplasia
F. Thrombosis
G. Myoma
H. Wart
I. Myxedema
J. Stricture
K. Ectopic
L. Wilm's
M. Dermoid cyst
N. Meckel's diverticulum
O. Anopsia
P. Adhesion
Q. Septicemia
R. Multiple myeloma
S. Epstein–Barr
T. Sarcoma
U. Condyloma latum
V. Goiter
W. Etiology
X. Histoplasmosis
Y. Cellulitis

_____ 1. Hypothyroidism in the adult
_____ 2. Local contraction of a tubular structure
_____ 3. Abnormal joining of parts to each other
_____ 4. Defect of vision
_____ 5. Malignant neoplasm of plasma cells
_____ 6. Virus that causes infectious mononucleosis
_____ 7. Opening between the left & right sides of the heart
_____ 8. Tubular outpouching from the distal ileum
_____ 9. Pathogenic bacteria in the blood
_____ 10. State of being sticky or thick
_____ 11. Lung disease due to inhalation of rock dust
_____ 12. Enlargement of the thyroid gland
_____ 13. Benign tumor of epithelial cells
_____ 14. Cause of a disease
_____ 15. Malignant renal tumor of infants & children
_____ 16. Type of dwarfism
_____ 17. Benign tumor projection from an epithelial surface
_____ 18. Formation of a clot in an unbroken blood vessel
_____ 19. Pregnancy occurring outside the endometrial cavity
_____ 20. Benign uterine smooth muscle tumor
_____ 21. Malignant tumor from connective and supportive tissues
_____ 22. Sexually transmitted warty tumor
_____ 23. Infection caused by a fungus
_____ 24. Inflammation involving skin or deeper tissue
_____ 25. Common benign cystic teratoma in the ovary

Answer Key	Notes
1. T	
2. J	
3. P	
4. O	
5. R	
6. S	
7. B	
8. N	
9. Q	
10. D	
11. A	
12. V	
13. H	
14. W	
15. L	
16. E	
17. C	
18. F	
19. K	
20. G	
21. T	
22. U	
23. X	
24. Y	
25. M	

Exercise 4-14 Anatomical Terms and Conditions

DIRECTIONS: Use each answer only once.

A. Flaccid
B. Parkinson's disease
C. Necrosis
D. Hyperemia
E. Menopause
F. Neonatal
G. Malaise
H. Polycythemia
I. Hyperventilation
J. Polyuria
K. Otitis media
L. Intubation
M. Postpartum
N. Myasthenia
O. Prosthesis
P. Invagination
Q. Sciatica
R. Micturition
S. In vivo
T. Hyperthermia
U. Shingles
V. Pyrexia
W. Incontinence
X. Prolapse
Y. Lactation

_____ 1. Excessive production of urine
_____ 2. Feeling of discomfort and uneasiness
_____ 3. Pertaining to the first 4 weeks after birth
_____ 4. Weakness of skeletal muscles
_____ 5. Act of expelling urine
_____ 6. Acute inflammation of the middle ear cavity
_____ 7. Artificial device to replace a body part
_____ 8. One part of a structure telescopes into another part
_____ 9. Termination of menstrual cycle
_____ 10. In the living body
_____ 11. Excess of blood in an area or part of the body
_____ 12. Condition in which temperature is above normal
_____ 13. Lacking muscle tone
_____ 14. Death of a cell or group of cells
_____ 15. Insertion of a tube through the nose or mouth
_____ 16. Abnormal increase in RBCs
_____ 17. Secretion and ejection of milk from breast
_____ 18. Occurring after delivery of a baby
_____ 19 Inability to retain urine, semen, or feces
_____ 20. Involuntary tremors and muscle weakness
_____ 21. Dropping or falling down of an organ
_____ 22. Rapid respirations
_____ 23. Pain at back of thigh and inside of leg
_____ 24. Elevated body temperature
_____ 25. Acute infection of the peripheral nervous system

Answer Key	Notes
1. J	
2. G	
3. F	
4. N	
5. R	
6. K	
7. O	
8. P	
9. E	
10. S	
11. D	
12. V	
13. A	
14. C	
15. L	
16. H	
17. Y	
18. M	
19. W	
20. B	
21. X	
22. I	
23. Q	
24. T	
25. U	

Exercise 4-15 Left Hand and Wrist Diagram

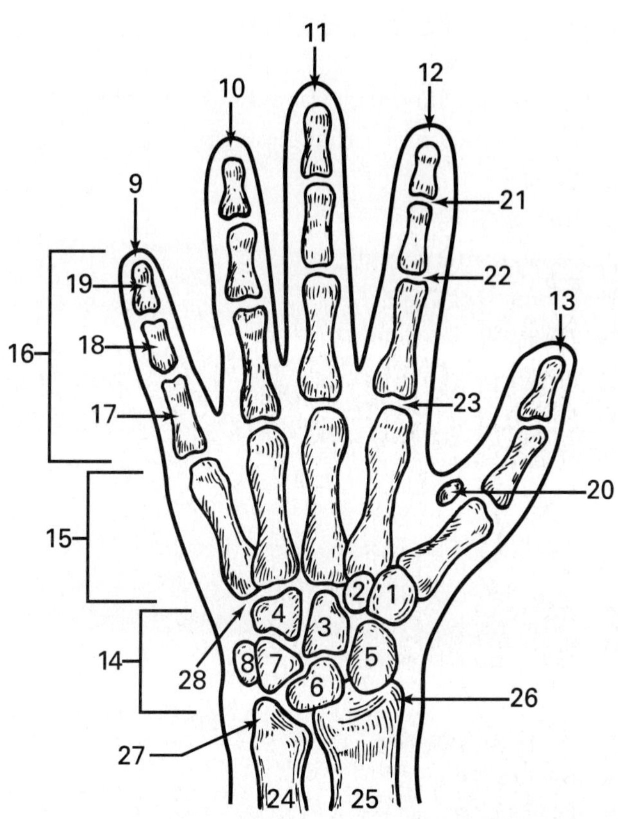

Plate 6 (Artwork courtesy of William F. Toeppe)

Plate 6. Left Hand and Wrist

Identify the structures labeled 1 to 28.

1.
2.
3.
4.
5.
6.
7.
8.
9.
10.
11.
12.
13.
14.
15.
16.
17.
18.
19.
20.
21.
22.
23.
24.
25.
26.
27.
28.

Plate 6. Left Hand and Wrist

1. Greater multangular (trapezium)
2. Lesser multangular (trapezoid)
3. Capitate
4. Hamate
5. Navicular (scaphoid)
6. Lunate (semilunar)
7. Triangular (triquetral)
8. Pisiform
9. Fifth digit
10. Fourth digit
11. Third digit
12. Second digit
13. First digit (thumb or pollex)
14. Carpal bones
15. Metacarpal bones
16. Phalanges
17. Proximal phalanx
18. Middle phalanx
19. Distal phalanx
20. Sesamoid bone
21. Distal Interphalangeal joint
22. Proximal interphalangeal joint
23. Metocarpophalangeal joint
24. Ulna
25. Radius
26. Styloid process of radius
27. Styloid process of ulna
28. Fifth carpometacarpal joint

Exercise 4-16 Finger, Hand, and Wrist Anatomy

DIRECTIONS: Answers may be used more than once.

A. Navicular
B. Diarthrodial
C. Tuft
D. Hamate
E. Pisiform
F. Phalanges
G. Greater multangular
H. Metacarpals
I. First digit
J. Styloid process
K. Capitate
L. Trapezoid
M. Triangular
N. Lunate
O. Fifth carpometacarpal joint
P. Third metacarpal
Q. Nine interphalangeal joints

_____ 1. Os magnum is also the _________
_____ 2. Medial carpal in proximal row
_____ 3. Triquetrum is also the _________
_____ 4. One hand contains 14 _________
_____ 5. Interphalangeal joints are of this type
_____ 6. Each hand contains five _________
_____ 7. Medial carpal in distal row
_____ 8. Carpal most commonly fractured
_____ 9. Radiocarpal joint
_____ 10. Scaphoid is also the _________
_____ 11. Distal ends of radius and ulna
_____ 12. Crown of distal phalanx
_____ 13. Lesser multangular is also the _________
_____ 14. Articulates with first metacarpal
_____ 15. Contains only two phalanges
_____ 16. Ulnar flexion demonstrates the _________
_____ 17. Second carpal in proximal row
_____ 18. Unciform is also the _________
_____ 19. Distal articulation with hamate
_____ 20. Distal articulation with capitate
_____ 21. Found on one hand relating to joints
_____ 22. Makes up the palm
_____ 23. Carpal articulating with thumb
_____ 24. Only carpal with just one name
_____ 25. Lies in close proximity to distal radius

Answer Key	Notes
1. K	
2. E	
3. M	
4. F	
5. B	
6. H	
7. D	
8. A	
9. B	
10. A	
11. J	
12. C	
13. L	
14. G	
15. I	
16. A	
17. N	
18. D	
19. O	
20. P	
21. Q	
22. H	
23. G	
24. E	
25. A	

Exercise 4-17 Right Radius and Ulna Diagram(Anterior View)

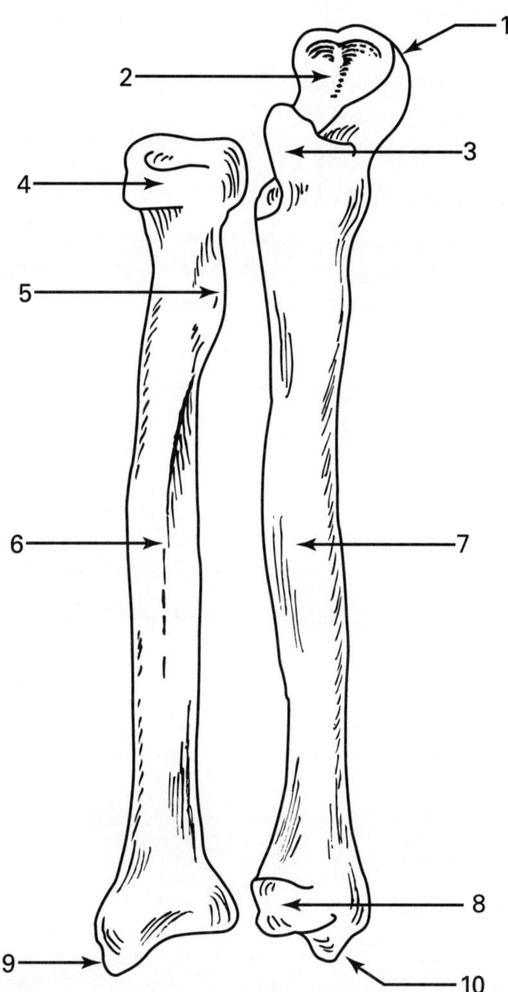

Plate 7 (Artwork courtesy of William F. Toeppe)

Plate 7. Right Radius and Ulna

Identify the structures labeled 1 to 10.

1.	6.
2.	7.
3.	8.
4.	9.
5.	10.

Plate 7. Right Radius and Ulna

1. Olecranon process
2. Semilunar notch
3. Coronoid process
4. Head of radius
5. Radial tuberosity
6. Shaft of radius
7. Shaft of ulna
8. Head of ulna
9. Styloid process of radius
10. Styloid process of ulna

Exercise 4-18 Left Humerus Diagram

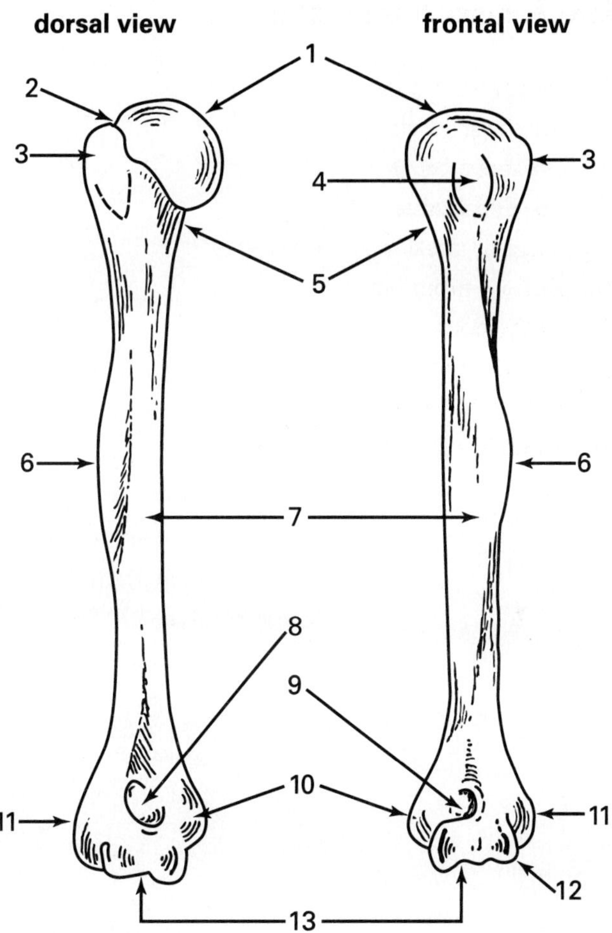

Plate 8 (Artwork courtesy of William F. Toeppe)

Plate 8. Left Humerus

Identify the structures labeled 1 to 13.

1.
2.
3.
4.
5.
6.
7.
8.
9.
10.
11.
12.
13.

Plate 8. Left Humerus

1. Head
2. Anatomic neck
3. Greater tubercle
4. Lesser tubercle
5. Surgical neck
6. Deltoid tuberosity
7. Shaft (body)
8. Olecranon fossa
9. Coronoid fossa
10. Medial epicondyle
11. Lateral epicondyle
12. Capitulum
13. Trochlea

Exercise 4-19 Forearm, Elbow, and Humerus Anatomy

DIRECTIONS: Answers may be used more than once.

A. Trochlea
B. Head of ulna
C. Neck of radius
D. Lateral epicondyle
E. Ulnar notch
F. Greater tuberosity
G. Medial epicondyle
H. Head of radius
I. Capitellum
J. Styloid processes
K. Radial notch
L. Olecranon and coronoid
M. Shaft
N. Radial tuberosity
O. Humeral condyle
P. Olecranon fossa
Q. Anatomical neck
R. Radial styloid process
S. Medial condyle
T. Semilunar notch
U. Ulna
V. Radius
W. Bicipital groove
X. Surgical neck

_____ 1. Slight constricted area below humeral head
_____ 2. Beaklike processes on proximal ulna
_____ 3. Cap over head of radius
_____ 4. Large bone of forearm
_____ 5. Located on distal radius and ulna
_____ 6. Shallow depression on lateral proximal ulna
_____ 7. Deep posterior depression on distal humerus
_____ 8. Large prominence on humerus proximal to the trochlea
_____ 9. Rough oval process on medial radius
_____ 10. Small projection on lateral distal humerus
_____ 11. Concave depression on proximal ulna
_____ 12. Located near the wrist above styloid
_____ 13. Fits into head of ulna
_____ 14. Tapered area below radial head
_____ 15. Large lateral process below anatomical neck
_____ 16. Small depression on medial aspect of distal radius
_____ 17. Depression located between the tuberosities
_____ 18. Located on medial humerus articulating with ulna
_____ 19. Lateral bone of forearm
_____ 20. Located near elbow joint at proximal end
_____ 21. Located midhumerus
_____ 22. Located at distal radius on thumb side
_____ 23. Located on lateral humerus articulating with head of radius
_____ 24. Tapered area below head and tuberosities
_____ 25. Entire distal end of the humerus

Answer Key	Notes
1. Q	
2. L	
3. I	
4. U	
5. J	
6. K	
7. P	
8. G	
9. N	
10. D	
11. T	
12. B	
13. E	
14. C	
15. F	
16. E	
17. W	
18. A	
19. V	
20. H	
21. M	
22. R	
23. I	
24. X	
25. O	

Exercise 4-20 Finger, Hand, and Wrist Positioning: Forearm, Elbow, and Humerus

DIRECTIONS: Answers may be used more than once.

A. Lateral elbow
B. Oblique position
C. Radial deviation
D. Semipronation
E. Proximal interplangeal joint
F. Midcarpal area
G. Digits 3 to 5
H. Lateral hand
I. AP elbow
J. First metacarpophalangeal joint
K. Coyle trauma position
L. Third metacarpophalangeal joint
M. Lateral forearm
N. Internal oblique
O. Postreduction wrist (wet cast)
P. AP projection of forearm
Q. Acute flexion
R. Gaynor–Hart
S. External oblique
T. External rotation of humerus
U. AP projection of humerus
V. Lateral transthoracic

_____ 1. Central ray to second metacarpophalangeal joint
_____ 2. Central ray location for PA wrist
_____ 3. Central ray location for thumb
_____ 4. Oblique position for wrist
_____ 5. 45 degrees oblique with lateral rotation
_____ 6. Central ray angled 20 degrees toward elbow
_____ 7. Central ray location for PA hand
_____ 8. Demonstrates all associated joints
_____ 9. Demonstrates radial head and neck region
_____ 10. Oblique position for hand
_____ 11. Central ray location for digits 2 to 5
_____ 12. Patient's arm rotated so thumb touches tabletop
_____ 13. Demonstrates coronoid process of ulna
_____ 14. Clearly demonstrates a profile of olecranon
_____ 15. Special projection for navicular
_____ 16. Central ray directed to anticubital space
_____ 17. Central ray midshaft with thumb up and elbow flexed 90 degrees
_____ 18. Demonstrates radial head and capitellum
_____ 19. Forearm supinated to include both joints
_____ 20. Central ray directed to surgical neck
_____ 21. Demonstrates greater tuberosity in profile
_____ 22. Best demonstrates olecranon fossa
_____ 23. Special projection for carpal canal
_____ 24. Trauma routine for proximal humerus
_____ 25. Increase mAs twofold and kV 10%

Answer Key

Notes

1. H
2. F
3. J
4. D
5. G
6. C
7. L
8. B
9. S
10. D
11. E
12. S
13. N
14. A
15. C
16. I
17. M
18. K
19. P
20. U
21. T
22. Q
23. R
24. V
25. O

Exercise 4-21 Chest Anatomy

DIRECTIONS: Use each answer only once.

A. Aorta
B. Cardiophrenic angle
C. Alveoli
D. Apex
E. Right lung
F. Pleura
G. Diaphragm
H. C6
I. Epiglottis
J. D4
K. Esophagus
L. Thymus gland
M. Carina
N. Mediastinum
O. Costophrenic angle
P. Pericardial sac
Q. Base
R. Uvula
S. Hilum
T. C5
U. Left lung
V. Thyroid cartilage
W. Fissure
X. Trachea
Y. Hemidiaphragm

_____ 1. Most inferior and lateral part of lung
_____ 2. Double-walled membrane covering of lung
_____ 3. Double-walled sac covering heart
_____ 4. Rounded upper area of lungs
_____ 5. Contains three lobes
_____ 6. Half of respiratory muscle
_____ 7. Temporary organ that disappears in adult
_____ 8. Back portion of soft palate
_____ 9. Ridge of lowest tracheal cartilage
_____ 10. Junction of larynx with trachea
_____ 11. Most inferior and medial part of lung
_____ 12. Posterior to trachea conveys food to stomach
_____ 13. Central area where bronchi meet lungs
_____ 14. Twenty C-shaped rings of cartilage
_____ 15. Largest artery in the body
_____ 16. Deep oblique canal dividing the lungs
_____ 17. Flap that prevents food and liquid from larynx
_____ 18. Adam's apple cartilage
_____ 19. Level of clavicles
_____ 20. Inferior concave area of each lung
_____ 21. Respiratory muscle
_____ 22. Space between the two lungs
_____ 23. Contains two lobes
_____ 24. Location of thyroid cartilage
_____ 25. Small air sacs and end of bronchi

Answer Key	Notes
1. O	
2. F	
3. P	
4. D	
5. E	
6. Y	
7. L	
8. R	
9. M	
10. H	
11. B	
12. K	
13. S	
14. X	
15. A	
16. W	
17. I	
18. V	
19. J	
20. Q	
21. G	
22. N	
23. U	
24. T	
25. C	

Exercise 4-22 Chest Positioning

DIRECTIONS: Use each answer only once.

A. Bucky
B. 90 degrees
C. 10 ribs
D. D6
E. Erect
F. Approximate PA chest technique
G. Autonomic
H. Decubitus
I. Left anterior oblique
J. 72-in. SID
K. Anterior oblique
L. Supine
M. Left lateral
N. Rotation (PA)
O. 50-in. SID
P. Apical lordotic
Q. True oblique
R. AP semierect
S. 7 ribs
T. 25 cm
U. Approximate lateral chest technique
V. Rotation (lateral)
W. Approximate mediastinal technique
X. Right lateral
Y. Base

_____ 1. Floor of each lung above diaphragm
_____ 2. Require tube to be angled so that film is perpendicular to central ray
_____ 3. Angle view of chest to remove superimposed clavicles
_____ 4. PA measures 20 lateral 30 cm true oblique = __________
_____ 5. 60 degrees oblique for heart size
_____ 6. 200 mA 1/30 sec 70 kV for 20 cm at 72 in.
_____ 7. Central ray location for PA chest
_____ 8. Minimum number superimposed on lungs (child)
_____ 9. Causes a distortion of heart and lungs
_____ 10. True lateral position of patient
_____ 11. Type of motion that is uncontrollable
_____ 12. Minimal number superimposed on lungs (adult)
_____ 13. +10 kV from PA on adult
_____ 14. 200 mA ½ sec 70 kV for 20 cm at 40-in. grid
_____ 15. Taken for air–fluid levels
_____ 16. Taken for pathology on right side
_____ 17. 40-in. chest with grid for mediastinum
_____ 18. Least desirable projection of chest
_____ 19. Appearance of posterior ribs
_____ 20. 200 mA 1/15 sec 90 kV for 30 cm at 72 in.
_____ 21. Taken for air fluid when unable to do erect
_____ 22. 45 degrees oblique for heart size
_____ 23. Asymmetrical appearance of SC joints
_____ 24. Gives an image of actual heart and lung size
_____ 25. Lateral position for heart size

Answer Key	Notes
1. Y	
2. R	
3. P	
4. T	
5. I	
6. F	
7. D	
8. S	
9. O	
10. B	
11. G	
12. C	
13. Q	
14. W	
15. E	
16. X	
17. A	
18. L	
19. V	
20. U	
21. H	
22. Q	
23. N	
24. J	
25. M	

Exercise 4-23 Right Foot

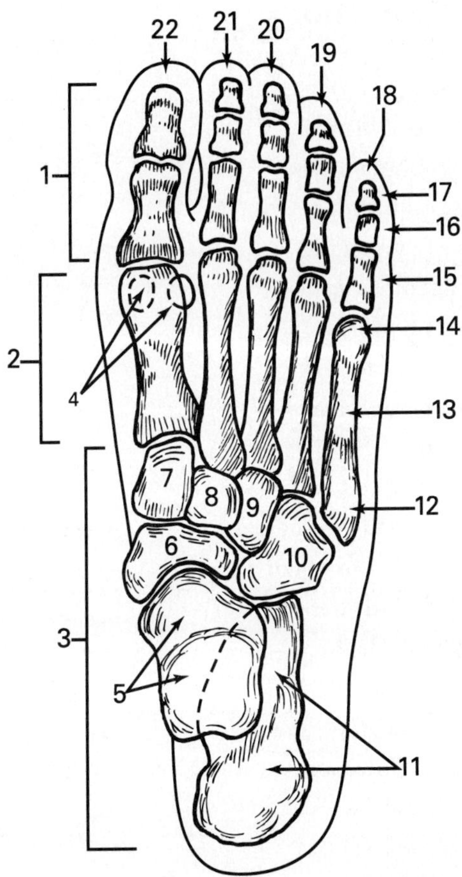

Plate 9 (Artwork courtesy of William F. Toeppe)

Plate 9. Right Foot

Identify the structures labeled 1 to 22.

1.
2.
3.
4.
5.
6.
7.
8.
9.
10.
11.
12.
13.
14.
15.
16.
17.
18.
19.
20.
21.
22.
23.

Plate 9. Right Foot

1. Phalanges
2. Metatarsal bones
3. Tarsal bones
4. Sesamoid bones
5. Talus (astragalus)
6. Navicular (scaphoid)
7. First cuneiform
8. Second cuneiform
9. Third cuneiform
10. Cuboid
11. Calcaneus (os calcis)
12. Base of fifth metatarsal
13. Shaft of fifth metatarsal
14. Head of fifth metatarsal
15. Proximal phalanx
16. Middle phalanx
17. Distal phalanx
18. Fifth or little toe
19. Fourth toe
20. Third toe
21. Second toe
22. First or great toe (hallux)

Exercise 4-24 Anatomy and Positioning of Foot, Ankle, and Calcaneus

DIRECTIONS: Use each answer only once.

A. Subtalar
B. 9
C. Cuboid
D. Lateral malleolus
E. Metatarsals
F. 40 degrees lateral oblique
G. Plantar
H. Os calcis
I. Interphalangeal joint
J. 26
K. Mediolateral
L. Astragalus
M. 5 to 15
N. Sesamoids
O. Diarthrodial joint
P. 7
Q. 45 degrees medial oblique
R. Longitudinal arch
S. Intermalleolar
T. Base
U. Third metatarsal
V. Medial malleolus
W. Inversion
X. 40-degree angle
Y. Distal first metatarsal

_____ 1. Tarsal found on lateral side of foot
_____ 2. Oblique position for fourth and fifth digits
_____ 3. Plane parallel to film for AP ankle
_____ 4. Central ray location for dorsoplantar foot
_____ 5. Small detached bones of foot
_____ 6. Location of sesamoid bones
_____ 7. Joint located between talus and calcaneus
_____ 8. Number of interphalangeal joints on foot
_____ 9. Oblique position for first, second, and third toe
_____ 10. Another name for talus
_____ 11. Number of tarsals
_____ 12. Foot 90 degrees with fifth metatarsal touching cassette
_____ 13. Largest of tarsal bones
_____ 14. Ankle joint is a hinge or __________
_____ 15. Total number of bones in foot and ankle
_____ 16. Expanded end of tibia
_____ 17. Expanded proximal end of each metatarsal
_____ 18. Referring to sole of foot
_____ 19. Make up instep of foot
_____ 20. Inward turning of the ankle
_____ 21. Springy curve composed of a medial and lateral part
_____ 22. Internal rotation of AP ankle
_____ 23. Expanded distal end of fibula
_____ 24. Calcaneus plantodorsal projection
_____ 25. Central ray for lateral toe

Answer Key	Notes
1. C	
2. F	
3. S	
4. U	
5. N	
6. Y	
7. A	
8. B	
9. Q	
10. L	
11. P	
12. K	
13. H	
14. O	
15. J	
16. V	
17. T	
18. G	
19. E	
20. W	
21. R	
22. M	
23. D	
24. X	
25. I	

Exercise 4-25 Right Tibia and Fibula Diagram (Anterior View)

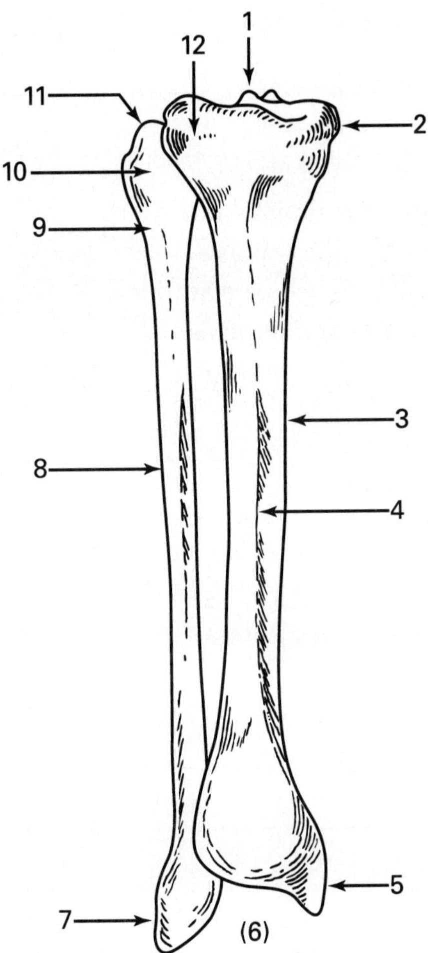

Plate 10 (Artwork courtesy of William F. Toeppe)

Plate 10. Right Tibula and Fibula

Identify the structures labeled 1 to 12.

1.
2.
3.
4.
5.
6.
7.
8.
9.
10.
11.
12.

Plate 10. Right Tibula and Fibula

1. Intercondylar eminence (spine)
2. Medial condyle of the tibia
3. Body or shaft of tibia
4. Anterior crest of tibia
5. Medial malleolus of tibia
6. Position occupied by talus bone
7. Lateral malleolus of fibula
8. Body or shaft of fibula
9. Neck of fibula
10. Head of fibula
11. Styloid process of fibula
12. Lateral condyle of tibia

Exercise 4-26 Left Femur Diagram

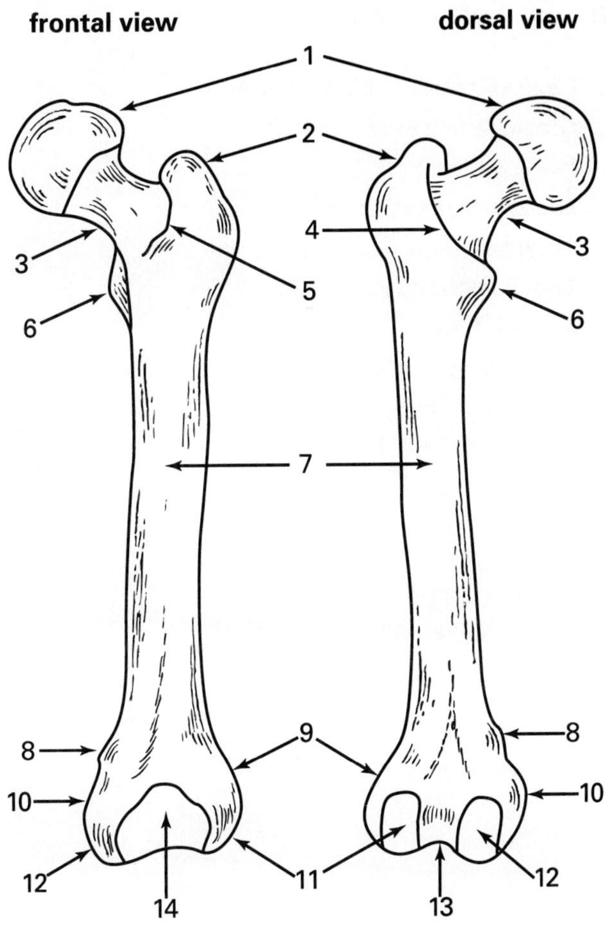

Plate 11 (Artwork courtesy of William F. Toeppe)

Plate 11. Left Femur

Identify the structures labeled 1 to 14.

1.	8.
2.	9.
3.	10.
4.	11.
5.	12.
6.	13.
7.	14.

Plate 11. Left Femur

1. Head of femur
2. Greater trochanter
3. Neck
4. Intertrochanteric crest
5. Intertrochanteric line
6. Lesser trochanter
7. Shaft of femur
8. Adductor tubercle
9. Lateral epicondyle
10. Medial epicondyle
11. Lateral condyle
12. Medial condyle
13. Intercondylar notch
14. Patellar surface

Exercise 4-27 Anatomy and Positioning of Tibia, Fibula, Knee, and Femur

DIRECTIONS: Answers may be used more than once.

A Menisci
B. Styloid process
C. Tibial plateau
D. Intertrochanteric crest
E. Femur
F. Patellar surface
G. Tunnel
H. Patella
I. Neck
J. Medial oblique
K. Lesser trochanter
L. Diaphysis
M. Epicondyles
N. Tibial spine
O. AP knee
P Osgood–Schlatter
Q. Popliteal
R. Tibial tuberosity
S. Intercondylar fossa
T. Base
U. Medial malleolus
V. Axial patella

_____ 1. Another name for shaft of fibula
_____ 2. Muscles attached at distal medial and lateral femur
_____ 3. Also called the intercondyloid eminence
_____ 4. Constricted segment of femur distal to head
_____ 5. Position not performed for vertical patella fracture
_____ 6. Separation of tibial tuberosity from shaft
_____ 7. Settegast, sunrise, or skyline
_____ 8. Helps to form ankle mortise
_____ 9. Ridge of bone between two trochanters posteriorly
_____ 10. Upper articular surface of tibial condyles
_____ 11. Extreme proximal head of fibula
_____ 12. Two cartilaginous pads in knee
_____ 13. Rough prominence on midanterior tibia
_____ 14. Space between femur and patella
_____ 15. Largest sesamoid bone
_____ 16. Semiaxial PA projection
_____ 17. Small prominence of femur located posteriorly and medial
_____ 18. Demonstrates proximal tibiofibular joint
_____ 19. Area directly posterior to knee joint
_____ 20. Tapered area of fibula below head
_____ 21. Notch located primarily on posterior femur
_____ 22. CR 5 degrees through knee joint
_____ 23. Strongest and longest bone in body
_____ 24. Position to demonstrate intercondyloid fossa
_____ 25. Most superior part of patella

Answer Key	Notes
1. L	
2. M	
3. N	
4. I	
5. V	
6. P	
7. V	
8. U	
9. D	
10. C	
11. B	
12. A	
13. R	
14. F	
15. H	
16. G	
17. K	
18. J	
19. Q	
20. I	
21. S	
22. O	
23. E	
24. G	
25. T	

Exercise 4-28 Pelvis Diagram

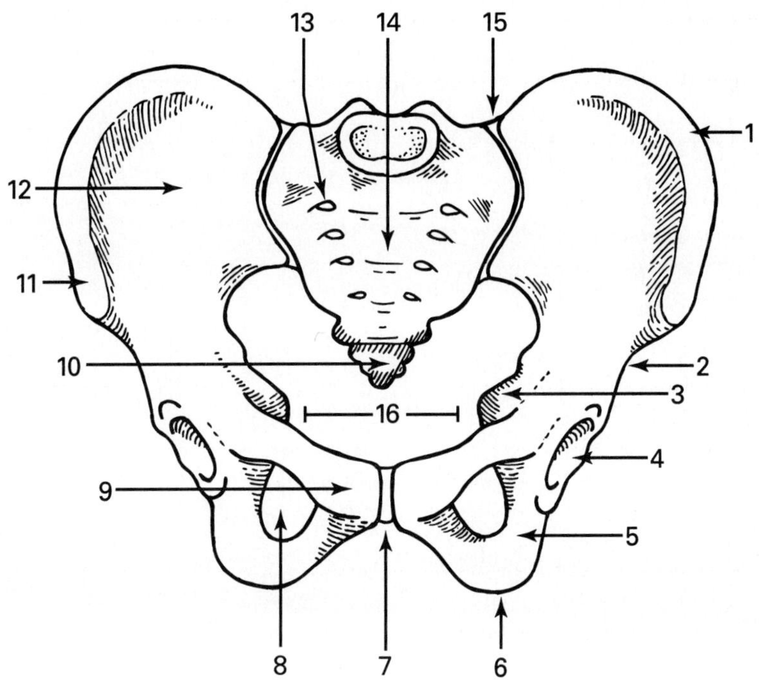

Plate 12 (Artwork courtesy of William F. Toeppe)

Plate 12. Pelvis

Identify the structures labeled 1 to 16.

1.	9.
2.	10.
3.	11.
4.	12.
5.	13.
6.	14.
7.	15.
8.	16.

Plate 12. Pelvis

1. Iliac crest
2. Anterior inferior iliac spine
3. Ischial spine
4. Acetabulum
5. Ischium
6. Ischial tuberosity
7. Symphysis pubis
8. Obturator foramen
9. Pubic bone
10. Coccyx
11. Anterior superior iliac spine
12. Ilium
13. Anterior sacral foramen
14. Sacrum
15. Sacroiliac joint

Exercise 4-29 Anatomy and Positioning of the Abdomen

DIRECTIONS: Use each answer only once.

A. Pyloric antrum
B. ASIS
C. Left lateral decubitus
D. Fundus
E. Iliac crest
F. Descending
G. Ischial tuberosities
H. Cecum
I. Axilla
J. Splenic
K. Psoas
L. Haustra
M. Duodenum
N. Ileum
O. Xiphoid process
P. Erect
Q. Symphysis pubis
R. Sigmoid
S. Greater trochanter
T. Appendix
U. Diaphragm
V. Pancreas
W. Rugae
X. Hepatic
Y. Jejunum

_____ 1. Right colic flexure
_____ 2. Part of small intestine following duodenum
_____ 3. Anterior junction of two pubic bones
_____ 4. Located directly above rectum
_____ 5. Position used when erect is not possible
_____ 6. Landmark: corresponds to level of symphysis
_____ 7. Located in C loop of duodenum
_____ 8. Inferior segment of stomach
_____ 9. Preferred position to demonstrate air–fluid levels
_____ 10. Top of film level for scout
_____ 11. Saclike folds of colon
_____ 12. Sac attached to posteromedial aspect of the cecum
_____ 13. Part located at anterior end of iliac crest
_____ 14. Saclike area below ileocecal valve
_____ 15. Separates thoracic from abdominal cavity
_____ 16. Major abdominal muscle
_____ 17. Left colic flexure
_____ 18. Top of film level for erect abdomen
_____ 19. Distal three-fifths of small intestine
_____ 20. First part of small intestine
_____ 21. Center of cassette for scout
_____ 22. Longitudinal stomach folds
_____ 23. Body prominences that bear weight of trunk when sitting
_____ 24. Area between transverse and sigmoid colon
_____ 25. Superior portion of stomach

Answer Key	Notes
1. X	
2. Y	
3. Q	
4. R	
5. C	
6. S	
7. V	
8. A	
9. P	
10. O	
11. L	
12. T	
13. B	
14. H	
15. U	
16. K	
17. J	
18. I	
19. N	
20. M	
21. E	
22. W	
23. G	
24. F	
25. D	

Exercise 4-30 Digestive System Diagram

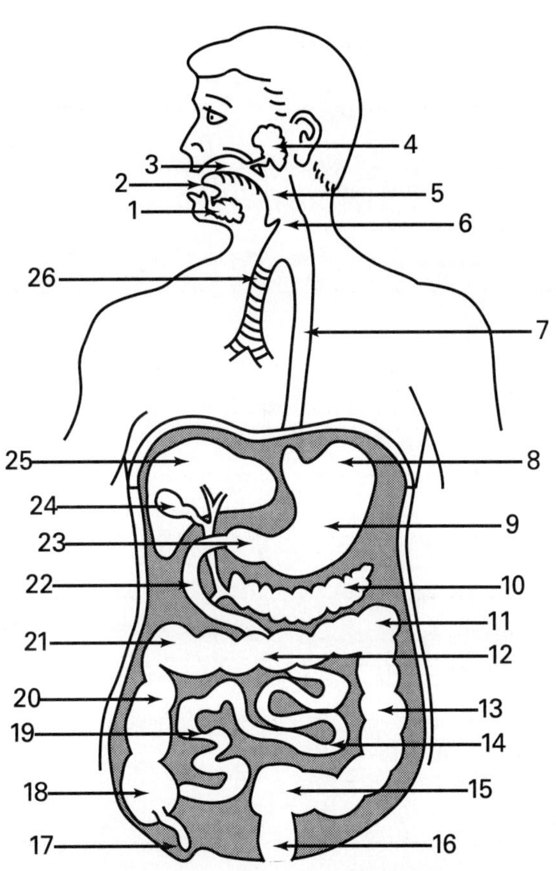

Plate 13 (Artwork courtesy of William F. Toeppe)

Plate 13. Digestive System

Identify the structures labeled 1 to 26.

1.
2.
3.
4.
5.
6.
7.
8.
9.
10.
11.
12.
13.
14.
15.
16.
17.
18.
19.
20.
21.
22.
23.
24.
25.
26.

Plate 13. Digestive System

1. Sublingual salivary gland
2. Tongue
3. Mouth or oral cavity
4. Parotid salivary gland
5. Oropharynx
6. Epiglottis
7. Esophagus
8. Fundus of the stomach
9. Body of the stomach
10. Pancreas
11. Splenic flexure
12. Transverse colon
13. Descending colon
14. Jejunum
15. Sigmoid colon
16. Rectum
17. Vermiform appendix
18. Cecum
19. Ileum
20. Ascending colon
21. Hepatic flexure
22. Duodenum
23. Pylorus of stomach
24. Gallbladder
25. Liver
26. Trachea

Exercise 4-31 Digestive System

DIRECTIONS: Use each answer only once.

A. Esophageal hiatus
B. Peritoneum
C. Buccal
D. Gastroenterology
E. Fundus
F. Mesocolon
G. Serosa
H. Ileocecal sphincter
I. Soft palate
J. Cirrhosis
K. Gastroesophageal
L. Mucosa
M. Cholecystokinin
N. Pylorus
O. Retroperitoneal
P. Hemorrhoids
Q. Greater omentum
R. Jejunum
S. Pepsin
T. Ascites
U. Mesentary
V. Uvula
W. Bilirubin
X. Villi
Y. Ulcer

_____ 1. Enzyme primary for digestion
_____ 2. Craterlike lesion in a membrane
_____ 3. Inner lining of the gastrointestinal tract
_____ 4. Principal bile pigment
_____ 5. Outermost layer of most of gastrointestinal canal
_____ 6. Glands that secrete small amounts of saliva
_____ 7. Organs lying on the posterior abdominal wall
_____ 8. Point where esophagus pierces diaphragm
_____ 9. Rounded portion of stomach left of the cardia
_____ 10. Study of stomach and intestines
_____ 11. Forms posterior portion of the roof of the mouth
_____ 12. Double fold of peritoneum connecting organs to posterior abdominal wall
_____ 13. Double-walled membrane of abdomen
_____ 14. Approximately 8 ft long and extends to ileum
_____ 15. Binds large intestine to posterior body wall
_____ 16. Hangs from free border of soft palate
_____ 17. Accumulation of serous fluid
_____ 18. Inhibits secretion of gastric juice
_____ 19. Opening from the ileum into large intestine
_____ 20. Four-layered apron fold over front of intestine
_____ 21. Scarred liver as a result of chronic inflammation
_____ 22. Sphincter that relaxes during swallowing
_____ 23. Projections of mucosa to increase absorption
_____ 24. Last division of stomach
_____ 25. Varicosities of the rectal veins

Answer Key	Notes
1. S	
2. Y	
3. L	
4. W	
5. G	
6. C	
7. O	
8. A	
9. E	
10. D	
11. I	
12. U	
13. B	
14. R	
15. F	
16. V	
17. T	
18. M	
19. H	
20. Q	
21. J	
22. K	
23. X	
24. N	
25. P	

Exercise 4-32 Gastrointestinal Tract

DIRECTIONS: Use each answer only once.

A. Chyme
B. Enzymes
C. Mastication
D. Pancreas
E. Paired cavities
F. Ligament of Treitz
G. Eustachian
H. Pharynx
I. T11
J. Esophagus
K. Hypersthenic
L. Salivary glands
M. Buccal cavity
N. Esophageal hiatus
O. Sthenic
P. Deglutition
Q. Cardiac antrum
R. Bulb or cap
S. Pharyngeal structures
T. Bile
U. T10
V. Peristalsis
W. Descending
X. Angular notch
Y. Asthenic

_____ 1. Distally, the pharynx continues as the _________
_____ 2. Massive type of body build
_____ 3. Esophagus terminates at _________
_____ 4. Longest segment of duodenum
_____ 5. Mouth connects posteriorly to _________ cavity
_____ 6. Aid to digestion manufactured in liver
_____ 7. Act of swallowing
_____ 8. Churned stomach contents
_____ 9. Propharynx and nasopharynx
_____ 10. Movement of chewing
_____ 11. Opening in diaphragm where esophagus passes
_____ 12. Lies in close relationship to duodenum
_____ 13. Nasal and tympanic cavities
_____ 14. 2-cm abdominal segment of esophagus
_____ 15. Another name for the oral cavity
_____ 16. Junction of duodenum and remainder of small bowel
_____ 17. Middle ear connects to the nasopharynx
_____ 18. Wavelike muscular contractions
_____ 19. Secretes saliva into the mouth
_____ 20. The incisura angularis is also _________
_____ 21. Biochemical catalysts that speed up digestion
_____ 22. Esophagus pierces diaphragm at _________
_____ 23. First part of small intestine
_____ 24. Very slender body type
_____ 25. Most common type of body build

Answer Key	Notes
1. J	
2. K	
3. I	
4. W	
5. H	
6. T	
7. P	
8. A	
9. S	
10. C	
11. N	
12. D	
13. E	
14. Q	
15. M	
16. F	
17. G	
18. V	
19. L	
20. X	
21. B	
22. U	
23. R	
24. Y	
25. O	

Exercise 4-33 Gastrointestinal Tract

DIRECTIONS: Use each answer only once.

A. Erect
B. L2
C. Edison
D. Small intestine
E. T6
F. Large bowel
G. Gastrografin
H. Fundus
I. Mueller
J. Hyposthenic
K. Transverse
L. Left anterior oblique (LAO)
M. Greater curvature
N. Pyloric sphincter
O. Valsalva
P. Cardiac notch
Q. AP Trendelenburg
R. Emulsification
S. LPO
T. Hydrometer
U. L4–L5
V. Left upper quadrant (LUQ)
W. PA and right anterior oblique (RAO)
X. L1
Y. Suspension

_____ 1. Water-soluble gastrointestinal contrast agent
_____ 2. Upper ballooned portion of stomach
_____ 3. Demonstrate barium in body and pylorus
_____ 4. Stomach of hypersthenic body type
_____ 5. Require a 60 degree angle of patient for cardiac series
_____ 6. Central ray location for scout
_____ 7. Duodenal bulb is slightly to the right of __________
_____ 8. Maneuver where you try to inhale against a closed glottis
_____ 9. Opening of distal stomach into duodenum
_____ 10. Located between incisura angularis and pylorus
_____ 11. Holds major portion of stomach
_____ 12. Process: large fat particles change to small
_____ 13. Stores and eliminates feces
_____ 14. Demonstrates a hiatal hernia
_____ 15. Measures specific gravity of $BaSO_4$
_____ 16. Slender body build: approximately 35% of patients
_____ 17. Absorption primarily takes place
_____ 18. Mixture of barium sulfate and water
_____ 19. Central ray for left posterior oblique (LPO), upper gastrointestinal tract (UGI) level
_____ 20. Begin GI series on an ambulatory patient
_____ 21. Holding of breath and bearing down
_____ 22. First known fluoroscopist
_____ 23. Central ray location for PA barium swallow
_____ 24. Another name for incisura cardiaca
_____ 25. Demonstrates air in distal stomach and duodenum

Answer Key	Notes
1. G	
2. H	
3. W	
4. K	
5. L	
6. U	
7. B	
8. I	
9. N	
10. M	
11. V	
12. R	
13. F	
14. Q	
15. T	
16. J	
17. D	
18. Y	
19. X	
20. A	
21. O	
22. C	
23. E	
24. P	
25. S	

Exercise 4-34 Barium Enema

DIRECTIONS: Use each answer only once.

A. AP
B. Volvulus
C. Defecation
D. Polyps
E. Cecum
F. Postevacuation films
G. Intussusception
H. Splenic flexure
I. 1½ m
J. Chassard–Lapine
K. Reflux
L. Paralytic
M. Fluoroscopy
N. Appendix
O. Large bowel
P. Gastrografin
Q. Sigmoid colon
R. 3 to 5 cm
S. Ileus
T. Right posterior oblique (RPO)
U. Ileocecal valve
V. Lateral
W. Sims
X. LAO
Y. Castor oil

_____ 1. Positions that show colon's ability to expel barium
_____ 2. Emptying of the bowel
_____ 3. Rectal catheters are inflated under _________
_____ 4. Most common location for bowel carcinoma
_____ 5. Segment of bowel that is most superior
_____ 6. Position that best demonstrates splenic flexure
_____ 7. Intestinal obstruction
_____ 8. Pelvic colon is also the _________
_____ 9. Distance enema tip is inserted
_____ 10. Bowel does not propel contents forward
_____ 11. Contrast medium used for perforations
_____ 12. Vermiform process
_____ 13. Demonstrates rectosigmoid area
_____ 14. Barium runs to here for completed barium enema
_____ 15. Twisting of the bowel
_____ 16. Backward flow
_____ 17. Length of colon
_____ 18. A barium enema with air demonstrates _________
_____ 19. Widest portion of the entire bowel
_____ 20. Position of patient for barium enema tip insert
_____ 21. Position often clips the left colic flexure
_____ 22. Telescoping one part of bowel to another
_____ 23. Demonstrates left half of large bowel
_____ 24. Irritant cathartic
_____ 25. Rectum is best demonstrated on a barium enema by _________

Answer Key	Notes
1. F	
2. C	
3. M	
4. O	
5. H	
6. T	
7. S	
8. Q	
9. R	
10. L	
11. P	
12. N	
13. J	
14. U	
15. B	
16. K	
17. I	
18. D	
19. E	
20. W	
21. A	
22. G	
23. X	
24. Y	
25. V	

Exercise 4-35 Gallbladder and Urinary Tract

DIRECTIONS: Use each answer only once.

A. Cortex
B. Fundus
C. Anterior
D. Common bile duct
E. Biliary calculi
F. Nephron
G. Urography
H. Cholografin
I. Common hepatic duct
J. Posterolateral
K. Sphincter of Oddi
L. Trigone
M. Cholecystography
N. Renal pelvis
O. Telepaque
P. Adipose capsule
Q. Bile
R. Urine
S. Cystic duct
T. Hypersthenic
U. Lithotomy
V. Cholecystogogue
W. Uremia
X. Prostate
Y. Micturation

_____ 1. Perirenal fat surrounding each kidney
_____ 2. Right and left hepatic ducts join to form the _________
_____ 3. Area where each ureter enters the bladder
_____ 4. Major function of gallbladder is to store _________
_____ 5. Gland surrounding the male urethra
_____ 6. Waste material formed by kidney
_____ 7. Radiographic exam of the gallbladder
_____ 8. Intravenous cholangiogram (IVC) contrast media
_____ 9. Broad inferior segment of gallbladder
_____ 10. Outer portion of each kidney
_____ 11. Gallbladder is located high in the _________
_____ 12. Common hepatic duct and cystic join to form _________
_____ 13. Common cholecystopaque
_____ 14. Gallstones or choleliths
_____ 15. Gallbladder and common bile duct connected by _________
_____ 16. Junction of ureter to major calyces
_____ 17. Fatty material: promotes gallbladder contraction
_____ 18. Gallbladder's location to ducts
_____ 19. Position for patient having a retrograde pyelogram
_____ 20. Buildup of nitrogenous wastes in blood
_____ 21. End of common bile duct muscle
_____ 22. Act of urinating
_____ 23. Functional unit of each kidney
_____ 24. Contrast-media examination of urinary system
_____ 25. Triangular area within the bladder

Answer Key	Notes
1. P	
2. I	
3. J	
4. Q	
5. X	
6. R	
7. M	
8. H	
9. B	
10. A	
11. T	
12. D	
13. O	
14. E	
15. S	
16. N	
17. V	
18. C	
19. U	
20. W	
21. K	
22. Y	
23. F	
24. G	
25. L	

Exercise 4-36 Skull Diagram (Frontal)

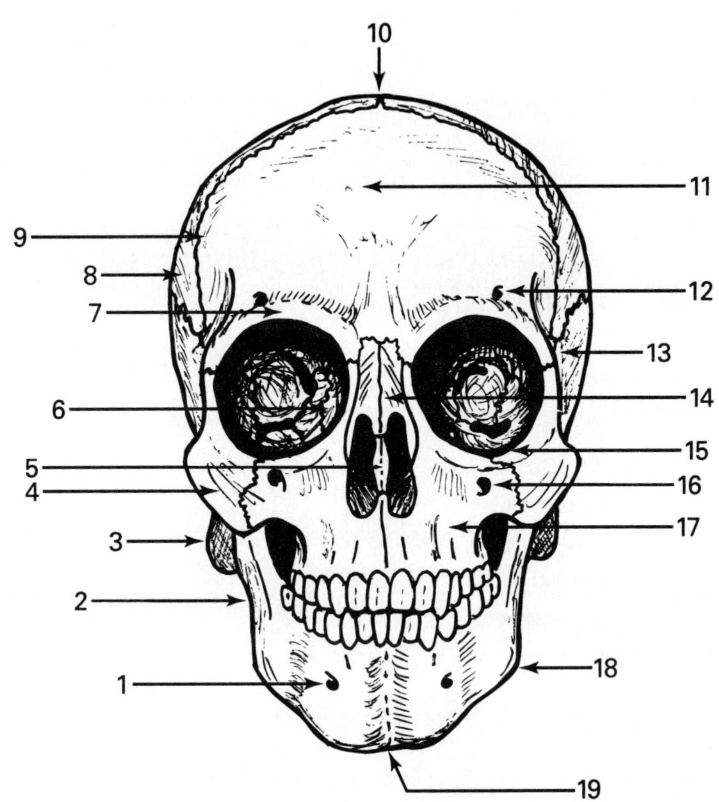

Plate 14 (Artwork courtesy of William F. Toeppe)

Plate 14. Skull (Frontal)

Identify the structures labeled 1 to 19.

1.
2.
3.
4.
5.
6.
7.
8.
9.
10.
11.
12.
13.
14.
15.
16.
17.
18.
19.

Plate 14. Skull (Frontal)

1. Mental foramen
2. Ramus of the mandible
3. Mastoid process of the temporal bone
4. Zygomatic bone
5. Nasal septum (volmer and perpendicular plate of ethmoid)
6. Lacrimal bone
7. Supraorbital margin
8. Parietal bone
9. Coronal suture
10. Sagittal suture
11. Frontal bone
12. Supraorbital foramen
13. Temporal bone
14. Nasal bone
15. Infraorbital margin
16. Infraorbital foramen
17. Maxilla
18. Angle of the mandible
19. Mandibular symphysis

Exercise 4-37 Skull Diagram (Lateral)

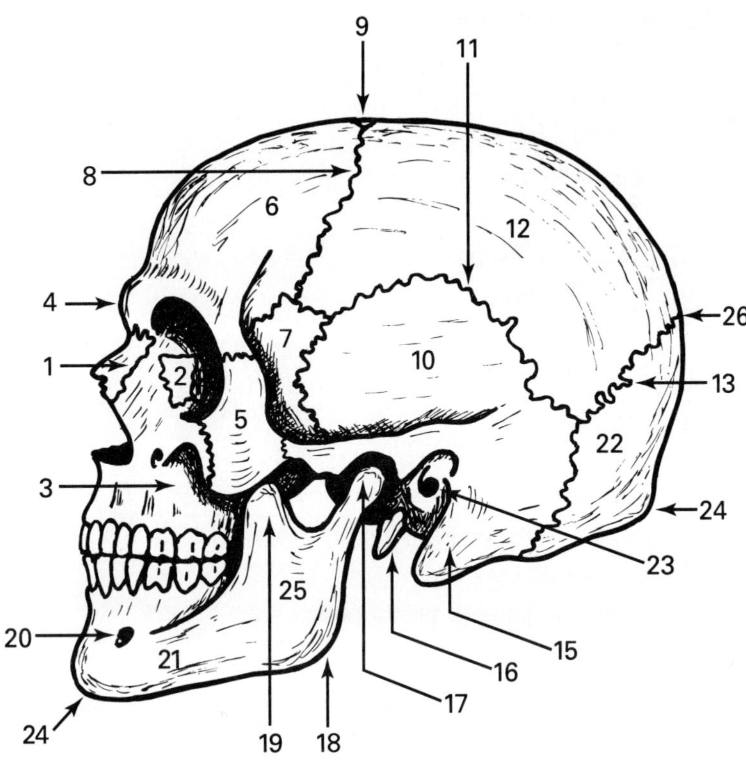

Plate 15 (Artwork courtesy of William F. Toeppe)

Plate 15. Skull (Lateral)

Identify the structures labeled 1 to 26.

1.
2.
3.
4.
5.
6.
7.
8.
9.
10.
11.
12.
13.
14.
15.
16.
17.
18.
19.
20.
21.
22.
23.
24.
25.
26.

Plate 15. Skull (Lateral)

1. Nasal bone
2. Lacrimal bone
3. Maxilla
4. Glabella
5. Zygomatic bone
6. Frontal bone
7. Sphenoid bone
8. Coronal suture
9. Bregma
10. Temporal bone
11. Squamosal suture
12. Parietal bone
13. Lambdoidal suture
14. External occipital protuberance
15. Mastoid process
16. Styloid process of temporal bone
17. Condylar process
18. Angle of the mandible
19. Coronoid process
20. Mental foramen
21. Body of the mandible
22. Occipital bone
23. External auditory (acoustic) meatus
24. Mental protuberance
25. Mandibular ramus
26. Lambda

Exercise 4-38 Cranial Anatomy

DIRECTIONS: Answers may be used more than once.

A. Parietal
B. Temporal
C. Occipital
D. Frontal
E. Ethmoid
F. Sphenoid

_____ 1. Holds the cribriform plate
_____ 2. Holds the labyrinths
_____ 3. Contains the external auditory meatus (EAM)
_____ 4. Contains the perpendicular plates
_____ 5. Contains the zygomatic process
_____ 6. Holds the styloid process
_____ 7. Contains the sella turcica
_____ 8. Holds the petrous pyramids
_____ 9. Holds the crista galli
_____ 10. Contains the turbinates
_____ 11. Holds the glabella
_____ 12. Holds the organs of hearing
_____ 13. Lies primarily on the floor of the skull
_____ 14. Contains the supraciliary arch
_____ 15. Contains the foramen magnum
_____ 16. Contains the squamous or vertical portion
_____ 17. Contains the lesser wings
_____ 18. Contains the orbital plate
_____ 19. Contains the inion or exterior occipital protuberance (EOP)
_____ 20. Forms the superior rim of the orbits
_____ 21. Forms most of the forehead
_____ 22. Holds eminences
_____ 23. Forms the roof of the cranium
_____ 24. Holds the dorsum sellae
_____ 25. Contains the greater wings

Answer Key | Notes

1. E
2. E
3. B
4. E
5. B
6. B
7. F
8. B
9. E
10. F
11. D
12. B
13. E
14. D
15. C
16. D
17. F
18. D
19. C
20. D
21. D
22. A
23. A
24. F
25. F

Exercise 4-39 Topographic Cranial Landmarks

DIRECTIONS: Use each answer only once.

A. Nasion
B. Lambda
C. Glabella
D. Gonion
E. Mental point
F. Squamous
G. Acanthion
H. Inion (EOP)
I. Top of ear attachment (TEA)
J. Pinna
K. Orbitomeatal line
L. Lambdoidal suture
M. Supraorbital groove
N. Squamosal
O. Bregma
P. Inner canthus
Q. Dorsum sellae
R. Infraorbital margin
S. Petrous pyramids
T. Sella turcica
U. Vertex
V. Pterygoids
W. Interpupillary line
X. Trempromandibular
Y. Clinoid processes

_____ 1. Anterior end of the sagittal suture
_____ 2. Vertical portion of the frontal bone
_____ 3. Four lateral and posterior flat processes on the sphenoid
_____ 4. Only diarthrodial joint of the skull
_____ 5. Bridge of nose between the eyebrows where frontal and nasal bones meet
_____ 6. Back wall of the saddle
_____ 7. Where the eyelids meet near the nose
_____ 8. Most superior part of the head
_____ 9. Smooth prominence between the eyebrows
_____ 10. Angle of the mandible
_____ 11. Corresponds to the level of the petrous ridge
_____ 12. Depression above the eyebrows
_____ 13. Most dense bone in the skull
_____ 14. Junction of the upper lip and nose
_____ 15. Central depression of the sphenoid
_____ 16. Inferior rim of the orbit
_____ 17. Separates the two parietals from the occipital
_____ 18. Triangle of the chin
_____ 19. Auricle of the ear
_____ 20. Line drawn between the pupils of the eye
_____ 21. Line between the outer canthus and EAM
_____ 22. Suture separating the parietals from the temporals
_____ 23. Depression at the bridge of the nose
_____ 24. Posterior end of the sagittal suture
_____ 25. Bump at the lower posterior cranium

Answer Key	Notes
1. O	
2. F	
3. Y	
4. X	
5. A	
6. Q	
7. P	
8. U	
9. C	
10. D	
11. I	
12. M	
13. S	
14. G	
15. T	
16. R	
17. L	
18. E	
19. J	
20. W	
21. K	
22. N	
23. A	
24. B	
25. H	

Exercise 4-40 Skull Positioning

DIRECTIONS: Answers may be used more than once. Items can require more than one answer.

A. Towne
B. PA Caldwell
C. Pirie (open mouth)
D. True PA skull
E. Modified Waters
F. True Caldwell
G. True Waters
H. Haas
I. Submentovertical (SMV)
J. Rhese
K. Lateral skull
L. Stenvers
M. Mayer
N. PA sella turcica
O. Schuller
P. Conedown–Sella lateral
Q. Law
R. PA mandible
S. Townes for mandible

_____ 1. Orbitomeatal line perpendicular to film, 25° angle cephalic
_____ 2. Rotate head 45° infraorbitomeatal line (IOML) perpendicular, 12° angle cephalic
_____ 3. Shows cranial base, foramen ovale and sphenoid sinus
_____ 4. IOML perpendicular to CR
_____ 5. Rotate head 45° IOML, parallel angle, 45° caudad
_____ 6. Interpupillary line perpendicular to film
_____ 7. Interpupillary lines perpendicular drop chin, 15° angle caudad
_____ 8. Mentomeatal line perpendicular to film
_____ 9. 30° angle caudad OML perpendicular to film
_____ 10. Rotate head 37° acanthomeatal line perpendicular to film
_____ 11. Orbitomeatal line perpendicular to film, 12° angle cephalic
_____ 12. Orbitomeatal line perpendicular to film, CR enters "below" foramen
_____ 13. 15 to 17° angle caudad OML perpendicular to film
_____ 14. Glabellomeatal line perpendicular to film, 23° angle caudad
_____ 15. CR enters ¾ in. anterior and superior from EAM
_____ 16. OML angle 37° to film
_____ 17. Interpupillary line perpendicular to film, 25° angle caudad
_____ 18. Shows maxillary sinus and facial bones
_____ 19. Petrous ridges projected lower half of maxillary sinus
_____ 20. Demonstrates mastoid's long axis and ossicles
_____ 21. Shows profile of mastoid and bony labyrinth
_____ 22. Places petrous ridges in lower third of orbit
_____ 23. Shows condyles, processes, and TM fossae
_____ 24. Demonstrate sphenoid sinus through mouth
_____ 25. Anterior and posterior clinoids superimposed

Answer Key

Notes

1. H
2. L
3. I
4. I
5. M
6. K/P
7. Q
8. C
9. A/S
10. J
11. N
12. R
13. B
14. F
15. P
16. G
17. O
18. G
19. E
20. M
21. L
22. F
23. S/A
24. C
25. P/K

Exercise **4-41 Facial Bones**

DIRECTIONS: Use each answer only once.

A. Waters
B. Alveolar
C. Nasion
D. Maxillary sinus
E. Maxillae
F. Rhese
G. Sphenoid strut
H. Palatine process
I. Basilar (SMV)
J. Base
K. Tripod
L. Malar
M. Nasion
N. Seven bones
O. Lacrimal
P. Nasofrontal suture
Q. Cleft palate
R. Axial
S. Optic foramen
T. Turbinates
U. Modified waters
V. Blowout
W. Deviated septum
X. Towne
Y. Acanthion

_____ 1. Three-point landing position for optic foramen
_____ 2. Congenital defect between palatines
_____ 3. Forms each orbit
_____ 4. Separates superior orbital fissure and optic canal
_____ 5. Process found on lower aspect of maxillae
_____ 6. Semiaxial AP projection for Zygomatic Arch
_____ 7. Optic nerve passes through the
_____ 8. CR exit point for Caldwell nasal bones
_____ 9. Large air-filled cavity in each maxillary bone
_____ 10. Demonstrate zygomatic arches bilaterally
_____ 11. Associated with the tear ducts
_____ 12. Central ray exit point for Waters
_____ 13. Forms upper jaw
_____ 14. Also known as "parietoacanthial projection"
_____ 15. Nasal area is pushed to one side, causing a, __________
_____ 16. Junction of the two nasal bones
_____ 17. Fracture along floor of orbit
_____ 18. Another name for the nasal conchae
_____ 19. Also known as "zygomatic bones"
_____ 20. Clearly demonstrated on lateral nasal film
_____ 21. Fracture involving zygomatic bone and its connections
_____ 22. Forms anterior roof of mouth
_____ 23. Projection taken with occlusal film for nose
_____ 24. Rim of the orbit
_____ 25. Clearly demonstrates floor of orbit

Answer Key

1. F
2. Q
3. N
4. G
5. B
6. X
7. S
8. M
9. D
10. I
11. O
12. Y
13. E
14. A
15. W
16. C
17. V
18. T
19. L
20. P
21. K
22. H
23. R
24. J
25. U

Notes

Exercise 4-42 Spinal Column Anatomy

DIRECTIONS: Use each answer only once.

A. Lamina
B. Atlantooccipital
C. Spinous process
D. Annulus fibrosus
E. Coccyx
F. Kyphosis
G. Atlantoepistropheal
H. 31
I. Bifid tip
J. Apex
K. 30 to 35-degree (angle) cephalic
L. L4–L5
M. "Scotty dogs"
N. Scioliosis
O. Spina bifida
P. Costotransverse joint
Q. Nucleus pulposus
R. Spondylolisthesis
S. Odontoid
T. 12
U. Intervertebral foramen
V. Epistropheus (axis)
W. Lateral mass
X. Apophysial joints
Y. Atlas

_____ 1. Vertebrae that have no body
_____ 2. Failure of two lamina to unite
_____ 3. Soft semigelatinous inner part of vertebrae
_____ 4. Double-forked tip
_____ 5. Sits laterally on each side of C1
_____ 6. Extends posteriorly from each pedicle
_____ 7. Most inferior point of sacrum
_____ 8. Tubercle of each rib articulates to form _________
_____ 9. Outer fibrous covering of vertebrae
_____ 10. Demonstrated in an oblique lumbar vertebra
_____ 11. Exaggerated humpback condition
_____ 12. Well demonstrated with a 10-degree caudad angle
_____ 13. Pairs of cranial nerves
_____ 14. Extends posteriorly from body to transverse process
_____ 15. Pairs of spinal nerves
_____ 16. Joint located between C1 and C2
_____ 17. AP L5–S1 tube direction
_____ 18. Abnormal lateral curvature
_____ 19. Toothlike prominence of C2
_____ 20. Another name for C2
_____ 21. Clearly demonstrated on cervical posterior oblique
_____ 22. Most posterior part of vertebrae
_____ 23. Forms 30- to 35-degree angle at iliac crest level
_____ 24. Anterior slippage of a vertebra
_____ 25. Joint between C1 and occipital bone

Answer Key

Notes

1. Y
2. O
3. Q
4. I
5. W
6. A
7. J
8. P
9. D
10. M
11. F
12. E
13. T
14. X
15. H
16. G
17. K
18. N
19. S
20. V
21. U
22. C
23. L
24. R
25. B

Exercise 4-43 Spinal Positioning

DIRECTIONS: Use each answer only once.

A. Cross table lateral
B. 5- to 8-degree angle
C. L3
D. Knees flexed
E. 45 degrees oblique
F. 15 degrees cephalad
G. Shows downside
H. T7
I. 35-degree angle
J. C4
K. Zygapophyseal joints
L. PA projection
M. Flexion
N. C7
O. 10 to 15 degrees caudad
P. 70 degrees oblique
Q. Shows upside zygapophyseal joints
R. Open mouth
S. Lateral
T. Extension
U. C3
V. Swimmers
W. D12
X. Chewing
Y. 20 degrees cephalad

_____ 1. Angle required for AP cervical
_____ 2. Demonstrate intervertebral foramina in the cervical spine
_____ 3. Gives best visualization of joint spaces
_____ 4. Projection required for C1 and C2
_____ 5. Frontal L5–S1 position requires __________
_____ 6. Patient sitting or standing looking up
_____ 7. RAO and LAO lumbar
_____ 8. When AP makes spinal column parallel to film
_____ 9. Level of film centering for AP lumbar
_____ 10. Level of gonion
_____ 11. Same level as top of shoulders
_____ 12. Angle required for AP sacrum projection
_____ 13. Special projection for lower cervical and upper dorsal
_____ 14. Demonstrates apophyseal joints
_____ 15. RPO and LPO lumbar
_____ 16. Special projection: blurs the mandible
_____ 17. Central ray location for AP thoracic
_____ 18. Angle required for AP coccyx projection
_____ 19. Projection required for trauma patients
_____ 20. Last set of ribs attached posteriorly
_____ 21. Demonstrated by oblique thoracic
_____ 22. Central ray location for lateral cervical
_____ 23. Required if lumbar spine is not supported
_____ 24. Patient sitting or standing looking down
_____ 25. Degree of rotational oblique for thoracic apophyseal joints

Answer Key	Notes
1. Y	
2. E	
3. L	
4. R	
5. I	
6. T	
7. Q	
8. D	
9. C	
10. U	
11. N	
12. F	
13. V	
14. S	
15. G	
16. X	
17. H	
18. O	
19. A	
20. W	
21. K	
22. J	
23. B	
24. M	
25. P	

Exercise **4-44** # Heart and Great Vessels Diagram

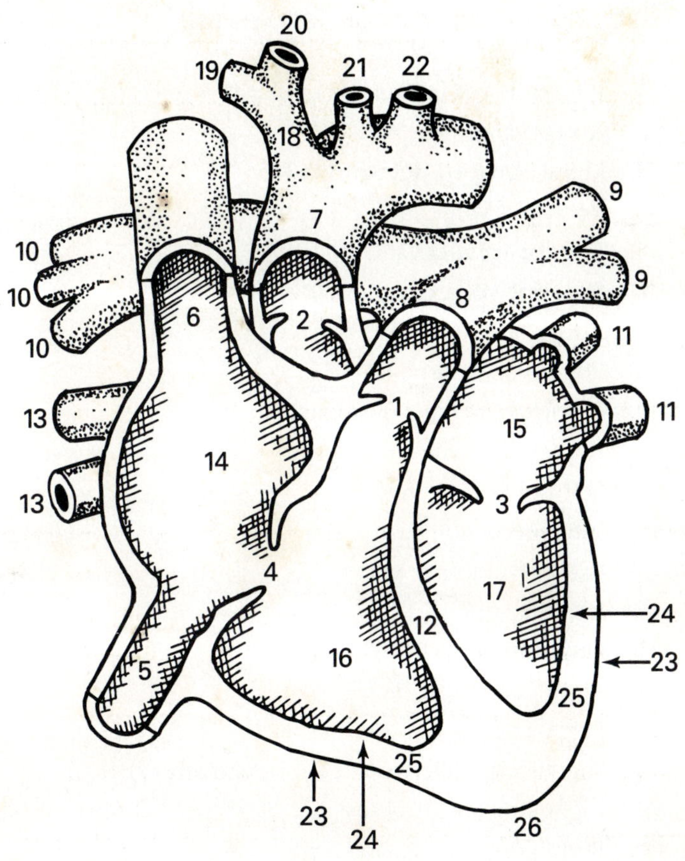

Plate 16 (Artwork courtesy of William F. Toeppe)

Plate 16. Heart and Great Vessels

Identify the structures labeled 1 to 26.

1.
2.
3.
4.
5.
6.
7.
8.
9.
10.
11.
12.
13.
14.
15.
16.
17.
18.
19.
20.
21.
22.
23.
24.
25.
26.

Plate 16. Heart and Great Vessels

1. Pulmonic (pulmonary) semilunar valve
2. Aortic valve
3. Mitral valve or bicuspid valve
4. Tricuspid valve
5. Inferior vena cava
6. Superior vena cava
7. Aorta
8. Pulmonary artery
9. Branches of left pulmonary artery
10. Branches of right pulmonary artery
11. Left pulmonary veins
12. Interventricular septum
13. Right pulmonary veins
14. Right atrium
15. Left atrium
16. Right ventricle
17. Left ventricle
18. Brachiocephalic trunk (inominate artery)
19. Right subclavian artery
20. Right common carotid artery
21. Left common carotid artery
22. Left subclavian artery
23. Pericardium
24. Endocardium
25. Myocardium
26. Apex

Exercise 4-45 Circulatory System

DIRECTIONS: Use each answer only once.

A. Circle of Willis
B. Internal jugular veins
C. Brachial artery
D. Popliteals
E. Right and left common iliacs
F. Left subclavian artery
G. Azygos vein
H. Right vertebral
I. Right and left femorals
J. Brachiocephalic artery
K. Dorsalis pedis
L. Superior mesenteric artery
M. Medial and lateral plantars
N. Right common carotid artery
O. Aorta
P. Right and left renals
Q. Celiac artery
R. Left common carotid artery
S. Axillaries
T. Inferior mesenteric veins
U. Inferior phrenic arteries
V. Right and left subclavian veins
W. Hemiazygos
X. Hepatic
Y. Great saphenous vein

_____ 1. Distributes blood to small intestine and part of large
_____ 2. First branch off arch of aorta
_____ 3. Located at back of knee joint
_____ 4. Second branch off the aorta
_____ 5. Off brachiocephalic near right common carotid
_____ 6. Continuation of brachials and basilics
_____ 7. Branches into medial ulnar and lateral radial arteries
_____ 8. Distributes blood to undersurface of diaphragm
_____ 9. First visceral aortic branch below diaphragm
_____ 10. Formed by union of anterior cerebral arteries
_____ 11. Receives blood from the face and neck
_____ 12. Drains blood from portions of the colon
_____ 13. Passes upward into the neck
_____ 14. Supply blood to sole of foot
_____ 15. Vessel located at ankle joint
_____ 16. Inferior bifurcation of abdominal aorta
_____ 17. Veins that drain the liver
_____ 18. External iliacs inferiorly branch into __________
_____ 19. Front of vertebral column and slightly left of midline
_____ 20. Distributes blood to vessels of left upper extremity
_____ 21. Unites with internal jugulars to form brachiocephalic veins
_____ 22. Largest blood vessel in the body
_____ 23. Distributes blood to kidneys
_____ 24. Longest vein in the body
_____ 25. Lies in front of vertebral column slightly right of midline

Answer Key

1. L
2. J
3. D
4. R
5. H
6. S
7. C
8. U
9. Q
10. A
11. B
12. T
13. N
14. M
15. K
16. E
17. X
18. I
19. W
20. F
21. V
22. O
23. P
24. Y
25. G

Notes

Exercise 4-46 Heart

DIRECTIONS: Use each answer only once.

A. Base
B. Four Pulmonary veins
C. Sternocostal surface
D. Aortic semilunar
E. Apex
F. Tricuspid
G. Right and left atria
H. Inferior border
I. Semilunar
J. Right atrium
K. Infarct
L. Superior border
M. Pacemaker
N. Right and left ventricles
O. Endocardium
P. Right border
Q. Mitral
R. Ischemia
S. Myocardium
T. Right and left pulmonary artery
U. Atrial fibrillation
V. Ascending aorta
W. Coronary sinus
X. Congestive heart failure
Y. Arrhythmia

_____ 1. Valves that prevent blood from flowing back
_____ 2. Formed by both atria
_____ 3. Thin layer of tissue inside the myocardium
_____ 4. Valve located between left ventricle and aorta
_____ 5. Reduced O_2 supply which weakens cells
_____ 6. Projects superiorly, posteriorly, and to right
_____ 7. Receives blood from all parts of body except liver
_____ 8. Cardiac muscle tissue
_____ 9. Formed by the tip of the left ventricle
_____ 10. Valve between right atrium and right ventricle
_____ 11. Blood returns to the heart by way of _________
_____ 12 Asynchronous contraction of the atrial muscle
_____ 13. Formed by right ventricle and left atrium
_____ 14. The pulmonary trunk divides into the _________
_____ 15. Collects deoxygenated blood and empties into the right atrium
_____ 16. Two upper chambers of the heart
_____ 17. Term for "sinoatrial node"
_____ 18. Formed by the right atrium
_____ 19. Death of area of tissue from poor circulation
_____ 20. Two lower chambers of the heart
_____ 21. Heart is not capable of supplying O_2 demands
_____ 22. Formed by right ventricle and slightly by left ventricle
_____ 23. Abnormal or irregular heart rhythm
_____ 24. Valve located between left atrium and left ventricle
_____ 25. Blood passing into left ventricle is pumped to _________

Answer Key	Notes
1. I	
2. L	
3. O	
4. D	
5. R	
6. A	
7. J	
8. S	
9. E	
10. F	
11. B	
12. U	
13. C	
14. T	
15. W	
16. G	
17. M	
18. P	
19. K	
20. N	
21. X	
22. H	
23. Y	
24. Q	
25. V	

Exercise 4-47 Patient Education (for Mammography)

DIRECTIONS: Use each answer only once.

A. LCIS (lobular carcinoma in situ)
B. Nulliparity
C. 40
D. Invasive ductal carcinoma (IDC), NOS
E. Lumpectomy
F. Greater than 5 cm in size
G. Increasing age
H. 0.8 rad
I. Invasive
J. Upper outer
K. Screening
L. Fibroadenoma
M. Diagnostic
N. Inflammatory carcinoma
O. Ultrasound
P. Radical mastectomy
Q. Up to 2 cm in size
R. 5000 rad
S. 50
T. 9
U. Metastatic
V. Needle aspiration
W. In situ
X. 2 to 5 cm in size
Y. Staging

_____ 1. Major risk factor for developing breast cancer
_____ 2. Quadrant in which most breast cancers occur
_____ 3. Special procedure to empty a cyst
_____ 4. Benign condition of the breast
_____ 5. Orange peel skin surface (peau d' orange)
_____ 6. Removal of entire breast, pectoral muscle, and lymph nodes
_____ 7. Hormonal risk factor for developing breast cancer
_____ 8. Baseline study should be done by age
_____ 9. Underarm lymph nodes are dissected for _________ purposes
_____ 10. Stage I breast cancer size
_____ 11. Pathology with risk to both breasts
_____ 12. 1 in _________ women will develop breast cancer
_____ 13. Maximum dose per breast (two views) per ACR guidelines
_____ 14. Disease that spreads to surrounding tissue
_____ 15. Removal of tumor and a small amount of surrounding tissue followed by radiation therapy
_____ 16. Type of mammogram done on symptomatic women
_____ 17. Annual mammograms should be done after age _________
_____ 18. Stage II breast cancer size
_____ 19. Radiation therapy total dose
_____ 20. Confined to the site of origin
_____ 21. Procedure used to differentiate cystic from solid lesions
_____ 22. Most common malignant condition of breast
_____ 23. Stage III breast cancer size
_____ 24. Type of mammogram done on asymptomatic women
_____ 25. Spread of primary tumor to other parts of body

Answer Key

Notes

1. G
2. J
3. V
4. L
5. N
6. P
7. B
8. C
9. Y
10. Q
11. A
12. T
13. H
14. I
15. E
16. M
17. S
18. X
19. R
20. W
21. O
22. D
23. F
24. K
25. U

Exercise 4-48 Clinical Breast Examination for Mammography

DIRECTIONS: Use each answer only once.

A. Malignant
B. Hard
C. 7.00
D. Lower outer quadrant (LOQ)
E. Access symmetry nipple parallel
F. Grid system
G. Circular
H. Upper outer quadrant (UOQ)
I. Benign
J. Flat middle three fingers
K. 10:00
L. Nipple
M. Medical history
N. Soft
O. Localization technique
P. Lying supine
Q. 2:00
R. Deep
S. Upper inner quadrant (UIQ)
T. Visual inspection
U. Search pattern
V. Palpation inspection
W. Parity
X. Lower inner quadrant (LIQ)
Y. Vertical strip

_____ 1. Upper outer quadrant (UOQ) on right is same as _________ o'clock
_____ 2. Part of visual inspection
_____ 3. Patient position for palpation technique
_____ 4. Looking for dimpling of skin is part of _________
_____ 5. Check for nipple discharge is part of _________
_____ 6. Method and technique of breast palpation
_____ 7. Current menstrual status is part of _________
_____ 8. 2:00 on left is same as _________
_____ 9. Name of a typical search pattern
_____ 10. On physical examination a malignant lump feels _________
_____ 11. Palpation pressure should be light, medium, and _________
_____ 12. Motion used for palpation
_____ 13. Lower inner quadrant (LIQ) on left is same as _________ o'clock
_____ 14. Poorly mobile lesion on physical exam is probably_________
_____ 15. Palpation should check the following areas of perimeter, axilla, and _________
_____ 16. Three patterns of search are circular, wedge, and _________
_____ 17. A freely mobile lesion on physical examination is most likely to be _________
_____ 18. 8:00 on the right is same as _________
_____ 19. 2:00 on the right is same as _________
_____ 20. Describing where abnormal findings are is part of _________
_____ 21. UOQ on left is same as _________ o'clock
_____ 22. A benign lump during examination would feel _________
_____ 23. Vertical strip pattern is part of _________
_____ 24. 7:00 on the left is the same as _________
_____ 25. Number of pregnancies is known as _________

Answer Key

Notes

1. K
2. E
3. P
4. T
5. V
6. J
7. M
8. H
9. F
10. B
11. R
12. G
13. C
14. A
15. L
16. Y
17. I
18. D
19. S
20. O
21. Q
22. N
23. U
24. X
25. W

Exercise

4-49 Breast Anatomy, Physiology, and Pathology

DIRECTIONS: Use each answer only once.

A. Cooper's ligaments
B. Fascia
C. Braline
D. Terminal Ductal Lobar Units (TDLUs)
E. Irregular
F. Same size
G. Clustered
H. UOQ
I. Involuation
J. less than 0.5 mm
K. Montgomery's tubercles
L. UIQ
M. Smooth
N. Axilla
O. Smaller
P. Gynecomastia
Q. Scattered
R. LIQ
S. Retromammary space
T. Greater than 2.0 mm
U. Tail of Spence
V. Estrogen
W. Fibroglandular
X. Fatty
Y. Juxtathorax

_____ 1. Thin layer of fat that separates breast from pectoral muscle
_____ 2. Benign enlargement of the male breast
_____ 3. Raised areas on the areolae
_____ 4. Margins of a benign lesion usually are _________
_____ 5. Thickest portion of the breast
_____ 6. Breast is enclosed in a membrane called _________
_____ 7. Base of the breast
_____ 8. Postmenopausal breast tissue usually will be _________
_____ 9. Axillary prolongation
_____ 10. Fibrous connective tissue
_____ 11. Radiographic size and size on palpation of a benign lesion will be _________
_____ 12. Radiographic size compared with size on palpation of a malignant lesion will be _________
_____ 13. Infra mammary fold (IMF) located at the _________
_____ 14. Stimulates growth of the breast
_____ 15. Malignant calcifications are typically _________
_____ 16. Ducts branch and end at _________
_____ 17. Young breast tissue
_____ 18. Decrease in glandular tissue
_____ 19. 15% of all lesions occur in the _________
_____ 20. Primary lymphatic drainage is to the
_____ 21. Margins of a malignant lesion usually are _________
_____ 22. Calcifications are distributed in this pattern for benign calcifications
_____ 23. Calcifications are distributed in this pattern for malignant calcifications
_____ 24. Benign calcifications are typically _________
_____ 25. 6% of all lesions occur in _________

Answer Key

1. S
2. P
3. K
4. M
5. H
6. B
7. Y
8. X
9. U
10. A
11. F
12. O
13. C
14. V
15. J
16. D
17. W
18. I
19. L
20. N
21. E
22. Q
23. G
24. T
25. R

Notes

Exercise 4-50 Positioning for Mammography

DIRECTIONS: Use each answer only once.

A. Elevate
B. Parallel
C. Craniocaudad
D. CV—cleavage
E. Tangential
F. Steeper
G. 90 degrees
H. Medial
I. FB (from below)
J. Exaggerated lateral cranio-caudad
K. Kyphotic
L. 60 degrees
M. Lateral and inferior
N. Rolled
O. 4
P. MLO
Q. Mediolateral oblique or MLO
R. Pectus excavatum
S. ML
T. AT—"Cleopatra"
U. Away
V. 180 degrees
W. Axillary tail
X. 8
Y. Shallower

_____ 1. View in which maximum amount of breast tissue is visualized
_____ 2. Average C-arm angle for mediolateral oblique (MLO) on a tall thin patient
_____ 3. Mobile borders of the breast are _________
_____ 4. For a superior lesion, a _________ view is also helpful
_____ 5. In concave view, the head turned _________
_____ 6. Good view for showing milk of calcium
_____ 7. Number of images for a routine study of both breasts
_____ 8. C-arm angle for forward-bending (FB) projection
_____ 9. Name for the two views that constitute a routine mammogram going superiorly to inferiorly
_____ 10. Name for the two views that constitute a routine mammogram going from UIQ to LOQ
_____ 11. Film is placed _________to pectoral muscle for MLO projection
_____ 12. Film is parallel to _________for AT view
_____ 13. Must be done with the IMF for proper positioning technique
_____ 14. MLO on short, stout patients requires a _________angle
_____ 15. View used to see tail of Spence
_____ 16. For a medial lesion, a _________ view is also helpful
_____ 17. View used to demonstrate skin calcifications
_____ 18. Number of images required for an implant study of both breasts
_____ 19. C-arm angle for an ML projection
_____ 20. MLO view on tall, thin patients requires a _________ angle
_____ 21. FB projection is very useful for _________ patients
_____ 22. For a far lateral lesion, a _________ view is also helpful
_____ 23. LMO projection is very useful for patients with _________
_____ 24. View used to separate superimposed tissue
_____ 25. For a superior lesion, a _________ view is also helpful

Answer Key

Notes

1. P
2. L
3. M
4. I
5. U
6. S
7. O
8. V
9. C
10. Q
11. B
12. W
13. A
14. Y
15. T
16. D
17. E
18. X
19. G
20. F
21. K
22. J
23. R
24. N
25. H

Exercise **4-51 Technical Application of Mammography**

DIRECTIONS: Use each answer only once.

A. Compression
B. Increased dose to the patient
C. 25 kVp
D. Photocell
E. 0.03 to 0.06 mm Mo
F. Molybdenum
G. 120 mAs
H. Reduce contrast
I. Phototiming
J. 300 mAs
K. Taut
L. Law of reciprocity fails
M. 0.03 to 0.037 mm Al
N. Crossover exposure
O. Reduces scatter
P. Source to image distance
Q. Star resolution pattern
R. Aluminum
S. Off-focus radiation
T. Inprove contrast
U. 22 kVp
V. Reduced dose to the patient
W. Beryllium
X. 0.1 to 0.2 mm
Y. 0.3 to 0.6mm

_____ 1. Easiest way to measure focal spot size
_____ 2. Use of grids
_____ 3. Disadvantage of using grids
_____ 4. Window and inherent filtration is _________
_____ 5. Reduces scatter radiation
_____ 6. Optimum kVp value for routine diagnostic imaging
_____ 7. Tube current for large focal spots should be _________
_____ 8. Source-to-image distance
_____ 9. Advantage of double screen/double emulsion film–screen system
_____ 10. Measured HVL should be _________
_____ 11. 15% increase in exposure is needed when _________
_____ 12. kVp value used for specimen radiography
_____ 13. You will _________ when compression is used
_____ 14. Anode target material
_____ 15. When using AEC, breast tissue must cover the _________
_____ 16. Size of focal spot for standard mammogram imaging
_____ 17. Compression should be done until _________
_____ 18. Size of focal spot for magnification imaging
_____ 19. Automatic exposure control is also known as _________
_____ 20. Molybdenum filter thickness in a mammographic x-ray tube
_____ 21. Disadvantage found when using double screen/double emulsion film–screen systems
_____ 22. Tube current for 0.1-mm focal spots should be _________
_____ 23. HVL is measured in units of _________
_____ 24. Use of high kVp value will _________
_____ 25. Collimation is used to prevent or limit _________

Answer Key	Notes
1. Q	
2. O	
3. B	
4. W	
5. A	
6. C	
7. J	
8. P	
9. V	
10. M	
11. L	
12. U	
13. T	
14. F	
15. D	
16. Y	
17. K	
18. X	
19. I	
20. E	
21. N	
22. G	
23. R	
24. H	
25. S	

Exercise 4-52 Mammographic Techniques

DIRECTIONS: Use each answer only once.

A. Low kVp value
B. Grid
C. OFD
D. Lowers
E. Scatter
F. Higher kVp value
G. Overlapping
H. Axilla
I. Magnification
J. Dense
K. Localized
L. Increased dose to patient
M. 0.1 mm
N. Unsharpness
O. Evaluate border of lesion
P. Spot
Q. Elevated
R. Air gap
S. Improve
T. Compressed
U. Motion
V. 22 kVp
W. Taut
X. Phototiming
Y. 0.3 mm

_____ 1. Spot compression is often combined with __________
_____ 2. Disadvantage when using grids
_____ 3. Focal spot size not used with magnification
_____ 4. Purpose of using magnification technique
_____ 5. Technique employed with magnification imaging
_____ 6. Spot compression is used to visualize __________ areas
_____ 7. Must be done with a specimen during imaging
_____ 8. Small focal spots are used with magnification because of the increased
_____ 9. Compression __________ dose
_____ 10. Exposure factor for fatty breasts will use __________
_____ 11. Grids __________ contrast
_____ 12. A magnification platform is __________
_____ 13. With spot compression, use __________ collimation
_____ 14. Compress the breast until __________
_____ 15. Type of breast for which grids are helpful
_____ 16. AEC
_____ 17. Focal spot size used with magnification imaging
_____ 18. Exposure factor for dense breasts will use __________
_____ 19. Never use a __________when performing magnification
_____ 20. Film markers are placed laterally by the __________
_____ 21. Typical kVp value used for specimen radiography
_____ 22. One reason for using compression: separates __________ structures
_____ 23. Second reason for using compression: reduces geometric __________
_____ 24 Third reason for using compression: reduces __________
_____ 25. Fourth reason for using compression: reduces __________ radiation

Answer Key	Notes
1. I	
2. L	
3. Y	
4. O	
5. R	
6. K	
7. T	
8. C	
9. D	
10. A	
11. S	
12. Q	
13. P	
14. W	
15. J	
16. X	
17. M	
18. F	
19. B	
20. H	
21. U	
22. G	
23. N	
24. U	
25. E	

Exercise **4-53** **Quality Assurance for Mammography**

DIRECTIONS: Use each answer only once.

A. Daily
B. Processing artifact
C. Lower
D. Film speed is increased
E. 2.20
F. Dedicated processing
G. Weekly
H. Sensitometer
I. Contrast index
J. 0.45
K. Monthly
L. 1.20
M. Film speed is reduced
N. Speed index
O. Higher
P. 5
Q. Quarterly
R. Film-handling artifact
S. 10
T. Extended processing
U. 0.02
V. Densitometer
W. 40
X. Semiannually
Y. Patient artifact

_____ 1. Film staying in developer longer with temperature remaining the same is known as _________

_____ 2. Cleaning of screens must be done _________

_____ 3. Instrument used to measure optical density

_____ 4. DD is the _________

_____ 5. Fixer retention test must be done _________

_____ 6. Minimum number of phantom images that must be seen

_____ 7. Low-volume processing requires _________ replenishment/sheet of film

_____ 8. Safelight fog should not exceed _________

_____ 9. Processor used to develop mammographic film only

_____ 10. Crescent marks on the film are a _________

_____ 11. If development time is decreased, _________

_____ 12. Instrument used to expose a sheet of film with a known quantity of light

_____ 13. Performing processor quality control must be done _________

_____ 14. Number of wires/inch for screen–film contact test tool

_____ 15. Film–screen contact test must be done _________

_____ 16. Stains on the film are a _________

_____ 17. Obtaining phantom images must be done _________

_____ 18. A good repeat film rate is _________

_____ 19. MD is the _________

_____ 20. High volume in processing requires _________ replenishment/sheet of film

_____ 21. MD on the sensitometric strip is step closest to _________

_____ 22. DD needs two readings; the first is to find the step closest to but not less than _________

_____ 23. Small white specks on the image in the axillary area usually are _________

_____ 24. If development time is increased, _________

_____ 25. DD needs two readings; the second is to find the step closest to but not over _________

Answer Key	Notes
1. T	
2. G	
3. V	
4. I	
5. Q	
6. S	
7. O	
8. U	
9. F	
10. R	
11. M	
12. H	
13. A	
14. W	
15. X	
16. B	
17. K	
18. P	
19. N	
20. C	
21. L	
22. J	
23. Y	
24. D	
25. E	

Exercise 4-54 Radiographic Procedures

Directions: Use each answer only once (CM=contrast media).

A. Invasive
B. Thermography
C. Isotopes
D. Pacemaker
E. Phlebogram (venogram)
F. Xeroradiography
G. Digital
H. Phototimer
I. Ciné
J. Echocardiography
K. Voiding cystourethrogram
L. MRI
M. Sinogram
N. Serial films
O. CAT scanning
P. Proctology
Q. Ultrasound
R. Arthroscopy
S. Ventriculogram
T. Orthodiagraphy
U. Noninvasive
V. T-tube cholangiogram
W. Biopsy
X. Lithotripsy
Y. Gynography

_____ 1. 6- to 10-day post operative check of bile drainage
_____ 2. Device that regulates density automatically
_____ 3. Breaking up a calculus with sound waves
_____ 4. Contrast media (CM) study of female reproductive organs
_____ 5. Spot films taken during barium study
_____ 6. Tracing of exact organ size
_____ 7. CM study of a tract in tissue
_____ 8. Motion pictures of an organ
_____ 9. Study of rectosigmoid area
_____ 10. Cross-sectional demonstration of anatomy
_____ 11. Technique for visualization of soft tissue
_____ 12. Visualization of joints with a scope
_____ 13. Study of organs with radioactive substances
_____ 14. Analysis of tissue samples
_____ 15. CM study of veins
_____ 16. Functional study of urethra and bladder
_____ 17. Procedure where skin is penetrated
_____ 18. Visualization of structures with sound waves
_____ 19. Study of structures by the heat they emit
_____ 20. Procedure using CM with ingestion or induction
_____ 21. Device that regulates heart rate
_____ 22. Subtraction of overlying anatomical structures
_____ 23. CM study of ventricles of brain
_____ 24. Visualization of structures by a magnetic field
_____ 25. Study of heart chambers and cardiofunction

Answer Key	Notes
1. V	
2. H	
3. X	
4. Y	
5. N	
6. T	
7. M	
8. I	
9. P	
10. O	
11. F	
12. R	
13. C	
14. W	
15. E	
16. K	
17. A	
18. Q	
19. B	
20. U	
21. D	
22. G	
23. S	
24. L	
25. J	

Exercise 4-55 Radiographic Procedures

DIRECTIONS: Use each answer only once.

A. Parotid gland
B. Elbow
C. Hypersthenic
D. PA axial
E. Fundus
F. Malaise
G. Transverse process
H. Colcher–Sussman
I. Metaphysis
J. Left lateral decubitus
K. Pinna
L. Meniscus
M. Capitullum
N. Sthenic
O. Apex
P. Maxilla
Q. Flat bones
R. Weight-bearing lateral
S. Pedicle
T. Bone marrow
U. Asthenic
V. Ligament of Treitz
W.. Extraoral
X Tragus
Y. Bregma

_____ 1. Extremely slender body build
_____ 2. Junction of duodenum with rest of small bowel
_____ 3. Demonstrate longitudinal arch of foot
_____ 4. Ribs, sternum, and scapula are _________
_____ 5. Also known as the anterior fontanel
_____ 6. Part of "scotty dog" that appears as the "eye"
_____ 7. Articulates with the head of the radius
_____ 8. Nasal spine is part of the _________
_____ 9. Located 1in. anterior inferior to the ear
_____ 10. Fat pad indicates a fractured _________
_____ 11. Projection that demonstrates the mentum
_____ 12. Most blood cells are produced within the _________
_____ 13. Part of the external structure of the ear
_____ 14. Demonstrates loose bodies of the knee
_____ 15. Gallbladder is higher and more to the right on this body type
_____ 16. Technique utilized for cephalo pelvimetry
_____ 17. "Nose" of the "scotty dog"
_____ 18. Half-moon-shaped knee cartilage
_____ 19. For a UGI the LPO show barium in the _________
_____ 20. Person with average physique
_____ 21. Distal part of the patella
_____ 22. Demonstrates pleural effusion
_____ 23. Vague feeling of body discomfort
_____ 24. Longitudinal growth of the long bone occurs
_____ 25. Flap of the ear

Answer Key	Notes
1. U	
2. V	
3. R	
4. Q	
5. Y	
6. S	
7. M	
8. P	
9. A	
10. B	
11. W	
12. T	
13. X	
14. D	
15. C	
16. H	
17. G	
18. L	
19. E	
20. N	
21. O	
22. J	
23. F	
24. I	
25. K	

Exercise **4-56 Radiographic Procedures**

DIRECTIONS: Use each answer only once (CM=contrast media).

A. Sialogram
B. Bronchography
C. Laryngogram
D. Angiography
E. Pelvimetry
F. Cholangiography
G. Mammography
H. Cystogram
I. Angiocardiography
J. Stereo radiography
K. Discography
L. Myelogram
M. Aortography
N. Pneumoencephalogram
O. Esophagram
P. Pyelogram
Q. Arthrogram
R. Teleroentgenogram
S. Hysterosalpingogram
T. Scanogram
U. Cholecystography
V. Lymphangiogram
W. Retrograde pyelogram
X. Urogram
Y. Tomography

_____ 1. Study of limb lengths
_____ 2. CM study of joints
_____ 3. CM study of the kidneys
_____ 4. CM study of the urinary tract
_____ 5. CM study of vertebral discs
_____ 6. Body section radiography
_____ 7. CM study of the lymphatic system
_____ 8. CM study of bile ducts
_____ 9. 6-ft standing chest
_____ 10. CM study of the urinary bladder
_____ 11. Study of kidney ureter/bladder (KUB) via a catheter
_____ 12. CM study of blood vessels
_____ 13. CM study of uterus and fallopian tubes
_____ 14. CM study of salivary glands
_____ 15. CM study of the aorta
_____ 16. Measurement of mother's pelvis and fetus
_____ 17. CM study of heart vessels
_____ 18. Study of breast tissue
_____ 19. CM study of the larynx
_____ 20. CM study of the gallbladder
_____ 21. CM study of the ventricles of the brain
_____ 22. CM study of bronchi and lungs
_____ 23. CM study of the spinal canal
_____ 24. Three-dimensional viewing of a structure
_____ 25. CM study of the esophagus

Answer Key

Notes

1. T
2. Q
3. P
4. X
5. K
6. Y
7. V
8. F
9. R
10. H
11. W
12. D
13. S
14. A
15. M
16. E
17. I
18. G
19. C
20. U
21. N
22. B
23. L
24. J
25. O

Exercise 4-57 Special Procedures

DIRECTIONS: Use each answer only once.

A. Xero radiography
B. Photographic subtraction
C. Film changers
D. Obturators
E. Burning sensation
F. Tolazoline
G. Seldinger Technique
H. Four-vessel angiogram
I. Knee arthography
J. Organic iodide salts
K. Vasovagal
L. Lidocaine
M. Time constraint
N. Guide wire
O. Positive contrast agent
P. Tourniquet
Q. Dilator
R. Tilt table
S. Three-vessel angiogram
T. Indicator dye
U. Meglumine salts
V. Lumbar
W. Atropine
X. Cisternal
Y. Venogram

_____ 1. Injection of carotids and left vertebral artery
_____ 2. Fits into catheter for placement
_____ 3. Drug used to lessen bradycardia during thoracic angiography
_____ 4. Cerebral angiography contrast media
_____ 5. Obstructs blood flow to superficial veins
_____ 6. Roll film, cassette, and cut film
_____ 7. Have less than 30% concentration
_____ 8. Used to enlarge the vessel
_____ 9. Consideration because _________ of absorption in arthography
_____ 10. Blunt tip needle inserts
_____ 11. Used to localize lymphatic vessels
_____ 12. Six-step catheter introduction
_____ 13. Preferred water-soluble contrast media
_____ 14. Administered to dilate vessels
_____ 15. Drug given to alleviate pain during injection
_____ 16. Response to fear
_____ 17. Waterless processing system
_____ 18. Normal feeling felt along injection pathway
_____ 19. Injection site for upper cervical pathology
_____ 20. Demonstrates lesions of the menisci
_____ 21. Both vertebral arteries are injected
_____ 22. Evaluates varicose veins
_____ 23. Injection at L2–L3
_____ 24. Cancels overlying structures
_____ 25. Required for myelography

Answer Key	Notes
1. S	
2. N	
3. W	
4. J	
5. P	
6. C	
7. O	
8. Q	
9. M	
10. D	
11. T	
12. G	
13. U	
14. F	
15. L	
16. K	
17. A	
18. E	
19. X	
20. I	
21. H	
22. Y	
23. V	
24. B	
25. R	

Exercise 4-58 Anatomy: Axial Skeleton Parts

DIRECTIONS: Answers may be used more than once.

A. Five
B. Twenty-four
C. Four
D. Three
E. Twelve
F. Thirty-one
G. Seven
H. Fourteen
I. Eight
J. Thirty-three
K. Six

_____ 1. Cuneiforms on one foot
_____ 2. Total number of styloids
_____ 3. Number of bones making up the calvarium
_____ 4. Pairs of cranial nerves
_____ 5. Number of carpals on one wrist
_____ 6. Ventricles of the brain
_____ 7. Phalanges on one hand
_____ 8. Number of paranasal sinuses pairs
_____ 9. Number of facial bones
_____ 10. Number of tarsals
_____ 11. Total number of fontanels
_____ 12. Parts of the duodenum
_____ 13. Bones making up cranium
_____ 14. Chambers in the heart
_____ 15. Cervical vertebrae
_____ 16. Sacral vertebra
_____ 17. Dorsal (thoracic) vertebrae
_____ 18. Number of carpals in proximal row
_____ 19. Metatarsals on one foot
_____ 20. Pairs of spinal nerves
_____ 21. Paired bones making up pelvis
_____ 22. Total number of vertebrae
_____ 23. Number of true ribs
_____ 24. Coccygeal vertebrae
_____ 25. Total number of ribs

Answer Key — Notes

1. D
2. K
3. C
4. E
5. I
6. C
7. H
8. C
9. H
10. G
11. K
12. C
13. I
14. C
15. G
16. A
17. E
18. C
19. A
20. F
21. D
22. J
23. G
24. C
25. B

Exercise 4-59 Eponyms

DIRECTIONS: Answers may be used more than once.

A. Cerebral arterial circle
B. Atrioventricular
C. Breast
D. Accessory duct
E. Submandibular
F. Pancreatic duct
G. Conduction
H. Glomerular capsule
I. Neurolemmocyte
J. Hepatopancreatic
K. Parotid
L. Paramesonephric
M. Thyroid cartilage
N. Sutural
O. Pancreatic islet
P. Vesicular ovarian
Q. Central
R. Uterine
S. Nephron
T. Bulbourethral
U. Rectouterine
V. Duodenal
W. Auditory
X. Intestinal gland

_____ 1. Bowman's gland
_____ 2. Graafian follicle
_____ 3. Duct of Santorini
_____ 4. Purkinje fiber
_____ 5. Ampulla of Vater
_____ 6. Adam's apple
_____ 7. Stensen's duct
_____ 8. Eustachian tube
_____ 9. Haversian canal
_____ 10. Cowper's gland
_____ 11. Crypt of Lieberkühn
_____ 12. Wormian bone
_____ 13. Bundle of His
_____ 14. Sphincter of Oddi
_____ 15. Cooper's ligament
_____ 16. Loop of Henle
_____ 17. Duct of Wirsung
_____ 18. Pouch of Douglas
_____ 19. Islets of Langerhans
_____ 20. Müller's duct
_____ 21. Fallopian tube
_____ 22. Brunner's gland
_____ 23. Wharton's duct
_____ 24. Circle of Willis
_____ 25. Schwann cell

Answer Key	Notes
1. H	
2. P	
3. D	
4. G	
5. J	
6. M	
7. K	
8. W	
9. Q	
10. T	
11. X	
12. N	
13. B	
14. J	
15. C	
16. S	
17. F	
18. U	
19. O	
20. L	
21. R	
22. V	
23. E	
24. A	
25. I	

Exercise 4-60 Projection Name to Body Part

DIRECTIONS: Answers may be used more than once.

A. Carpal canal
B. Acoustic ossicles
C. Cephalometry
D. Wrist
E. Cervical spine
F. Hip dislocation
G. Facial and sinuses
H. Knee (intercondyloid fossa)
I. Acromioclavicular articulation
J. Rectosigmoid
K. Atlantooccipital articulation
L. Sacroiliac motion
M. Acetabulum
N. Jugular foramina
O. Atlas and axis
P. Temporal styloid
Q. Knee arthrography
R. Femoral necks
S. Orbital fissure
T. Liver and spleen

_____ 1. Buetti method for __________
_____ 2. Alexander's method demonstrates the __________
_____ 3. Camp–coventry method for __________
_____ 4. Andren–Wehlins method for __________
_____ 5. Beclere method for __________
_____ 6. Chamberlin method for __________
_____ 7. Judet approach demonstrates the __________
_____ 8. Cahoon method for __________
_____ 9. Arcelin method for __________
_____ 10. Bertel method for __________
_____ 11. Colcher–Sussman method for __________
_____ 12. Andren–Von Rosen method for __________
_____ 13. Dorland–Fremont technique for __________
_____ 14. Burmans method for __________
_____ 15. Gaynor–Hart method for __________
_____ 16. Judd method for __________
_____ 17. Grandy method for __________
_____ 18. Caldwell method for __________
_____ 19. Ottonello method for __________
_____ 20. Benassi method for __________
_____ 21. Ball method for __________
_____ 22. Chassard–Lapine method for __________
_____ 23. Thoms method for __________
_____ 24. Chausse method for __________
_____ 25. Cleaves method for __________

Answer Key	Notes
1. K	
2. I	
3. H	
4. Q	
5. H	
6. L	
7. M	
8. P	
9. B	
10. S	
11. C	
12. F	
13. E	
14. D	
15. A	
16. O	
17. E	
18. G	
19. E	
20. T	
21. C	
22. J	
23. C	
24. N	
25. R	

Exercise 4-61 Projection Name to Body Part

DIRECTIONS: Answers may be used more than once.

A. Eye foreign bodies
B. Cranium
C. Facial bones
D. Mammography
E. Pneumothorax
F. Scoliosis
G. Frontal and ethmoidal sinuses
H. Shoulder
I. Elbow
J. Tarsals
K. Clubfoot
L. Nephrotomography
M. Optic foramen
N. Cranial base or mastoid
O. Dens
P. Femoral neck and hip
Q. Stomach
R. Pharynx

_____ 1. Ekimsky method for __________

_____ 2. Lilienfeld method for __________

_____ 3. Comberg method for __________

_____ 4. Caldwell method for __________

_____ 5. Lysholm method for __________

_____ 6. Sweet method for __________

_____ 7. Valdini method for __________

_____ 8. Conway–Cowell method for __________

_____ 9. Ferguson method for __________

_____ 10. Towne method for __________

_____ 11. Cleopatra position for __________

_____ 12. Waters method for __________

_____ 13. Haas method for __________

_____ 14. Dubilier–Monteith method for __________

_____ 15. Clements modification for __________

_____ 16. Vogt bone-free position for __________

_____ 17. Griswold method for __________

_____ 18. Leonard–George method for __________

_____ 19. Rhese method for __________

_____ 20. Fuchs method for __________

_____ 21. Law method for __________

_____ 22. Gugliantini method for __________

_____ 23. Gunson method for __________

_____ 24. Feist–Mankin method for __________

_____ 25. Gordon method for __________

Answer Key	Notes
1. E	
2. P	
3. A	
4. G	
5. N	
6. A	
7. B	
8. K	
9. F	
10. B	
11. D	
12. C	
13. B	
14. L	
15. H	
16. A	
17. I	
18. P	
19. M	
20. O	
21. C	
22. Q	
23. R	
24. J	
25. Q	

Exercise

4-62 Projection Name to Body Part

DIRECTIONS: Use each answer only once.

A. Radial head
B. Fifth lumbar
C. Knee
D. Sphenoid strut
E. Intervertebral Discs
F. Hand
G. Hypoglossal canal
H. Acoustic nerve
I. Salivary glands
J. Mastoid process
K. Clubfoot
L. Dens
M. Jugular foramina
N. Large intestine
O. Knee
P. Sinuses
Q. Lung
R. Sesamoid
S. Hip
T. Shoulder
U. Sternoclavicular
V. Temporal bone
W. Scapula
X. Clinoid process
Y. Carpal bridge

_____ 1. Holmblad method for _________
_____ 2. Kovacs method for _________
_____ 3. Norgaard method for _________
_____ 4. Kemp–Harper method for _________
_____ 5. Holly method for _________
_____ 6. Duncan–Hoen method for _________
_____ 7. Kite method for _________
_____ 8. Henschen method for _________
_____ 9. Kurzbauer method for _________
_____ 10. Hough method for _________
_____ 11. Welin technique for _________
_____ 12. Miller method for _________
_____ 13. Lawrence method for _________
_____ 14. Hickey method for _________
_____ 15. Kjellberg method for _________
_____ 16. Kasabach method for _________
_____ 17. Kuchendorf method for _________
_____ 18. Iglauer method for _________
_____ 19. Low–Beer method for _________
_____ 20. Lilienfeld method for _________
_____ 21. Lewis method for _________
_____ 22. Lysholm method for _________
_____ 23. Lentino method for _________
_____ 24. Mahoney method for _________
_____ 25. Lorenz method for _________

Answer Key	Notes
1. C	
2. B	
3. F	
4. M	
5. A	
6. E	
7. K	
8. H	
9. U	
10. D	
11. N	
12. G	
13. T	
14. J	
15. Q	
16. L	
17. O	
18. I	
19. V	
20. W	
21. R	
22. X	
23. Y	
24. P	
25. S	

Exercise 4-63 Projection Name to Body Part

DIRECTIONS: Answers may be used more than once.

A. Clavicle
B. Shoulder
C. Barium enema
D. Clubfoot
E. Sacroiliac joints
F. Trachea
G. Mastoid process
H. Patella
I. Zygomatic arch
J. Lung
K. Scapula
L. Metatarsophalangeals
M. Temporomandibular joints
N. Maxillary sinus
O. Temporal bone
P. Pelvic bones
Q. Prostate
R. Thoracic spine
S. Optic foramen

_____ 1. Settegast method for __________
_____ 2. Marzujian method for __________
_____ 3. Twining position for __________
_____ 4. Oppenheimer method for __________
_____ 5. McLaughlin method for __________
_____ 6. Waters method for __________
_____ 7 Rigler method for __________
_____ 8. Merchant method for __________
_____ 9. Marique method for __________
_____ 10. Hickey method for __________
_____ 11. Meese method for __________
_____ 12. May method for __________
_____ 13. Taylor method for __________
_____ 14. Alexander method for __________
_____ 15. Causton method for __________
_____ 16. Henschen method for __________
_____ 17. Blackett–Healy method for __________
_____ 18. Teufel method for __________
_____ 19. West Point method for __________
_____ 20. Miller method for __________
_____ 21. Sugiura–Hasegawa method for __________
_____ 22. Staunig method for __________
_____ 23. Pearson method for __________
_____ 24. Hirtz method for __________
_____ 25. Zanelli method for __________

Answer Key	Notes
1. H	
2. K	
3. F/R	
4. R	
5. A	
6. N	
7. J	
8. H	
9. D	
10. G/P	
11. E	
12. I	
13. P	
14. S	
15. L	
16. G	
17. B	
18. P	
19. B	
20. C	
21. Q	
22. P	
23. B	
24. O	
25. M	

Exercise 4-64 Position/Projection

DIRECTIONS: Answers may be used more than once.

A. 5 degrees cephalic
B. 30 degrees caudad
C. 40 degrees plantar
D. 15 degrees caudad
E. 35 degrees cephalic
F. 10 degrees toward heel
G. 25 degrees caudad
H. 40 degrees caudad
I. 12 degrees cephalic
J. 10 to 15 degrees cephalic
K. 12 degrees caudad
L. 10 degrees caudad
M. 20 degrees cephalic
N. 45 degrees cephalic

_____ 1. Anterior oblique of cervical spine
_____ 2. Axiolateral oblique mandible
_____ 3. AP knee
_____ 4. Lateral oblique for mammography
_____ 5. Tunnel knee
_____ 6. Proximal humerus (transthoracic)
_____ 7. Chassard–Lapine for rectosigmoid
_____ 8. Semiaxial AP for sella turcica
_____ 9. Dorsoplantor foot
_____ 10. AP sacrum
_____ 11. Caldwell position of cranium
_____ 12. Frontal (female) L5–S1 lumbar
_____ 13. AP semiaxial clavicle
_____ 14. Law position for temporomandibular joints
_____ 15. Occipital (Towne) position of cranium
_____ 16. Semiaxial calcaneus
_____ 17. AP coccyx
_____ 18. Semiaxial AP mandible
_____ 19. Frog leg position
_____ 20. Stenver's position for mastoids
_____ 21. Schuller's position for TMJs
_____ 22. Semiaxial AP for zygomatic arch
_____ 23. Arcelin position for petrous pyramids
_____ 24. Law position for mastoids
_____ 25. AP cervical spine

Answer Key	Notes
1. D	
2. E	
3. A	
4. H	
5. H	
6. J	
7. N	
8. B	
9. F	
10. J	
11. D	
12. E	
13. J	
14. D	
15. B	
16. C	
17. L	
18. B	
19. J	
20. I	
21. G	
22. B	
23. K	
24. D	
25. M	

Exercise 4-65 Anatomy to Patient Position

DIRECTIONS: Answers may be used more than once.

A. Transallary lateral
B. Dorsal decubitus
C. AP lordotic
D. Radial deviation
E. Erect
F. AP
G. RAO
H. Internal oblique
I. Lateral decubitus
J. External rotation
K. Semipronation
L. External oblique
M. Lateral
N. Bilateral weight bearing
O. Medial oblique
P. Internal rotation
Q. Translateral
R. SMV
S. Trendelenburg
T. RPO
U. Soft tissue lateral

_____ 1. Coronoid process of ulna
_____ 2. Common bile duct
_____ 3. Duodenum free of superimposition
_____ 4. Lumbar (downside) apophysial joints
_____ 5. Patellar surface
_____ 6. Umbilical hernias
_____ 7. Cervical apophysial joints
_____ 8. Relationship of humeral head and neck to glenoid
_____ 9. Cranial base and sphenoid sinus
_____ 10. Distal tibiofibular joint
_____ 11. Lung apices
_____ 12. Lateral view of femoral neck
_____ 13. Femoral heads, necks and greater trochanters
_____ 14. Air–fluid levels
_____ 15. Scaphoid without foreshortening
_____ 16. Small pleural effusions
_____ 17. Radial head and neck region
_____ 18. Demonstration of hiatial hernia
_____ 19. Wrist joints
_____ 20. Talus and subtalar joint
_____ 21. Greater tuberosity of humerus in profile
_____ 22. Frontal demonstration of radius and ulna
_____ 23. Demonstrates upper esophagus and trachea
_____ 24. Both AC joint spaces
_____ 25. Left axillary margin of ribs

Answer Key	Notes
1. H	
2. T	
3. G	
4. T	
5. M	
6. B	
7. M	
8. A	
9. R	
10. O	
11. C	
12. Q	
13. P	
14. E	
15. D	
16. I	
17. L	
18. S	
19. K	
20. M	
21. J	
22. F	
23. U	
24. N	
25. G	

Exercise 4-66 Pathology

DIRECTIONS: Use each answer only once.

A. Sequestrum
B. Exostosis
C. Gargoylism
D. Ankylosis
E. Spondylolisthesis
F. Sprengel's deformity
G. Contracture
H. Rickets
I. Acrania
J. Scurvy
K. Decalcification
L. Pulmonary edema
M. Spondylitis
N. Osteolysis
O. Paget's disease
P. Asthma
Q. Osgood–Schlatter disease
R. Craniostenosis
S. Legg–Calvé-Perthes disease
T. Dextro position
U. Embolus
V. Dysplasia
W. Fallot's tetralogy
X. Pneumothorax
Y. Atelectasis

_____ 1. Disease caused by calcium and vitamin D loss
_____ 2. Dissolution of bone from lesions
_____ 3. Congenital disorder of scapula
_____ 4. Inflammation of a vertebra
_____ 5. Abnormality of development
_____ 6. Bronchial disease caused by allergy
_____ 7. Growing disorder of the pelvis
_____ 8. Piece of dead bone separated from sound bone
_____ 9. Osteitis deformation of skeletal structure
_____ 10. Premature closure of sutures
_____ 11. Inflammation of tibial tubercle
_____ 12. Air in chest cavity outside lungs
_____ 13. Disease caused by deficient vitamin C
_____ 14. Partial or complete absence of cranium
_____ 15. Effusion of serous fluid to lungs
_____ 16. Bony outgrowth of bone
_____ 17. Displacement of organ to opposite side
_____ 18. Disease characterized by dwarfism
_____ 19. Abnormal joint immobility
_____ 20. Combination of four heart defects
_____ 21. Clot or plug formed from other material
_____ 22. Forward displacement of a vertebra on another
_____ 23. Pathologic shortening or shrinkage
_____ 24. Total or partial lung collapse
_____ 25. Loss of calcium salts from bones

Answer Key	Notes
1. H	
2. N	
3. F	
4. M	
5. V	
6. P	
7. S	
8. A	
9. O	
10. R	
11. Q	
12. X	
13. J	
14. I	
15. L	
16. B	
17. T	
18. C	
19. D	
20. W	
21. U	
22. E	
23. G	
24. Y	
25. K	

Exercise 4-67 Pathology

DIRECTIONS: Use each answer only once.

A. Iatrogrenic
B. Anthrocosis
C. Ureterocele
D. Cystadenoma
E. Achalasia
F. Osteoclasts
G. Leiomyoma
H. Pseudocyst
I. Bulla
J. Situs inversus
K. Osteophytes
L. Atheroma
M. Transposition
N. Enchondroma
O. Zenker's
P. Anencephaly
Q. Teratoma
R. Seminoma
S. Glioma
T. Subluxation
U. Involucrum
V. Spondylolysis
W. Nidus
X. Neoplastic
Y. Rickets

_____ 1. Osseous outgrowth (spur)
_____ 2. Large vesicle filled with air
_____ 3. Diverticulum located in pharyngoesophageal region
_____ 4. Congenital absence of the cranial vault
_____ 5. Displacement of a viscus to the opposite side
_____ 6. Mass of plaque occurring in atherosclerosis
_____ 7. Breaking down of the body of a vertebra
_____ 8. Adverse condition occurring from treatment
_____ 9. Cystlike dilation of the terminal ureter
_____ 10. Failure of lower esophageal sphincter to relax
_____ 11. Cells associated with absorption and removal of bone
_____ 12. Incomplete or partial dislocation
_____ 13. Adenoma associated with cystoma
_____ 14. Osteomalacia caused by deficiency of vitamin D
_____ 15. Area of sclerosis associated with osteoid osteoma
_____ 16. Excessive inhalation of coal dust
_____ 17. Reversal of thorax and abdominal viscera
_____ 18. Abnormal or displaced space resembling a cyst
_____ 19. Benign growth in the metaphysis
_____ 20. Neoplasm commonly found in the ovary or testis
_____ 21. Benign tumor derived from smooth muscle
_____ 22. Tumor occurring in cerebral hemispheres
_____ 23. New, abnormal tissue growth
_____ 24. Malignant neoplasm of the testis
_____ 25. Sheath of new bone surrounding necrosed bone

Answer Key

Notes

1. K
2. I
3. O
4. P
5. M
6. L
7. V
8. A
9. C
10. E
11. F
12. T
13. D
14. Y
15. W
16. B
17. J
18. H
19. N
20. Q
21. G
22. S
23. X
24. R
25. U

Exercise 4-68 Anatomical Terms and Conditions

DIRECTIONS: Use each answer only once.

A. Dystrophia
B. Alkalosis
C. Hemostasis
D. Acidosis
E. Bolus
F. Extravasation
G. Aerobic
H. Herniated
I. Aseptic
J. Scirrhous
K. Bright's disease
L. Gout
M. Adenoids
N. Gestation
O. Hirsutism
P. Enuresis
Q. Adhesion
R. Hodgkin's disease
S. Gavage
T. Ataxia
U. Verrucous
V. Down's syndrome
W. Dysphoria
X. Constipation
Y. Exudate

_____ 1. Excessive growth of hair in females and children
_____ 2. Pharyngeal tonsils
_____ 3. Glomerulonephritis
_____ 4. Free from infection
_____ 5. Involuntary discharge of urine
_____ 6. Lack of muscular coordination
_____ 7. Feeding through a tube
_____ 8. Blood pH is between 7.35 and 6.80
_____ 9. Sadness or hopelessness
_____ 10. Abnormal joining of parts to each other
_____ 11. Period of intrauterine fetal development
_____ 12. Soft, rounded mass of food
_____ 13. Resembling a wartlike growth
_____ 14. Blood pH is between 7.45 and 8.00
_____ 15. Infrequent or difficult defecation
_____ 16. Malignant disorder in lymph nodes
_____ 17. Defect with an extra copy of chromosome 21
_____ 18. Rupture of an intervertebral disc
_____ 19. Requiring molecular oxygen
_____ 20. Escaping fluid that oozes from a space
_____ 21. Escape of fluid from a vessel into the tissue
_____ 22. Acid crystals present in joints and kidneys
_____ 23. Progressive weakening of muscle
_____ 24. Stoppage of bleeding
_____ 25. Hard, densely packed tumors

Answer Key	Notes
1. O	
2. M	
3. K	
4. I	
5. P	
6. T	
7. S	
8. D	
9. W	
10. Q	
11. N	
12. E	
13. U	
14. B	
15. X	
16. R	
17. V	
18. H	
19. G	
20. Y	
21. F	
22. L	
23. A	
24. C	
25. J	

Exercise 4-69 Fractures

DIRECTIONS: Use each answer only once.

A. Fracture signs
B. Crepitus
C. Partial
D. Closed
E. Flap
F. Callus
G. Open reduction
H. Displaced
I. Trimalleolar
J. Postreduction
K. Boxers
L. T-fracture
M. Monteggia
N. March (stress)
O. Tripod
P. Torus
Q. Le Fort
R. Subluxation
S. Depressed
T. Complete
U. Fat pad sign
V. Closed reduction
W. Nonunion
X. Multiple
Y. Dislocation

_____ 1. Fracture of fifth metacarpal in hand
_____ 2. Bilateral and horizontal fractures of maxillae
_____ 3. Occurs in foot from excessive pressure
_____ 4. Fracture of proximal third of ulnar shaft
_____ 5. Both ends of bone (across) are broken
_____ 6. Healing does not occur and fragments do not join
_____ 7. Fracture in skull where line produces a flap
_____ 8. Bending in skull or facial area
_____ 9. Folding or pressure fracture
_____ 10. Edema, ecchymosis, deformity, and nerve injury
_____ 11. Anatomical alignment is poor
_____ 12. Slipping of bone under displacement
_____ 13. Fracture of zygomatic or malar bone
_____ 14. Fracture across bone is incomplete
_____ 15. Occurs above and across the condyles of a long bone
_____ 16. Growth of new bone tissue
_____ 17. Bone does not penetrate the skin
_____ 18. Three sides of ankle joint broken
_____ 19. Bone is out of joint; not in normal articulation
_____ 20. Repair of fracture by surgery
_____ 21. Act of realigning the fractured ends
_____ 22. Sound heard when rubbing fracture ends together
_____ 23. Nonvisualized underlying fracture of elbow
_____ 24. Repair of fracture alignment without incision
_____ 25. Bone is broken in a variety of places

Answer Key	Notes
1. K	
2. Q	
3. N	
4. M	
5. T	
6. W	
7. E	
8. S	
9. P	
10. A	
11. H	
12. R	
13. O	
14. C	
15. L	
16. F	
17. D	
18. I	
19. Y	
20. G	
21. J	
22. B	
23. U	
24. V	
25. X	

Exercise 4-70 Fractures

DIRECTIONS: Use each answer only once.

A. Greenstick
B. Buttonhole
C. Smith's
D. Compression
E. Oblique
F. Compound
G. Potts
H. Double
I. Linear
J. Bumper
K. Telescope
L. Comminuted
M. Spontaneous
N. Reverse Potts
O. Ununited
P. Colles
Q. Bennet's
R. Spiral
S. Simple
T. Avulsion
U. Contre coup
V. Blowout
W. Impacted
X. Intertrochanteric
Y. Stellate

_____ 1. Occurs from pathology
_____ 2. Occurs 5 in. above distal radius
_____ 3. Pedestrian occurs 2 in. distal to knee
_____ 4. Tearing of piece of bone attached to muscle
_____ 5. Break of long bone in spiral shape
_____ 6. Fracture of distal radius
_____ 7. Fracture at floor of orbit
_____ 8. Opposite side fracture
_____ 9. Occurs at distal tibia with splintering
_____ 10. Occurs in vertebrae, crushing of disc
_____ 11. Straight-line fracture
_____ 12. Object knocks hole in bone
_____ 13. Across femoral trochanters
_____ 14. Occurs at an angle other than horizontal over vertical
_____ 15. Bending fracture occurs in children (cartilage)
_____ 16. Noncomplicated fracture
_____ 17. One end driven into another
_____ 18. Broken in many pieces
_____ 19. One end is pushed into another
_____ 20. 3 in. above distal fibula
_____ 21. Penetrates skin
_____ 22. Fracture at proximal end of first metacarpal
_____ 23. Two fractures at two locations on one bone
_____ 24. Branch-type fracture in skull
_____ 25. No union or exostosis

Answer Key	Notes
1. M	
2. C	
3. J	
4. T	
5. R	
6. P	
7. V	
8. U	
9. N	
10. D	
11. I	
12. B	
13. X	
14. E	
15. A	
16. S	
17. W	
18. L	
19. K	
20. G	
21. F	
22. Q	
23. H	
24. Y	
25. O	

Section 5
Patient Care and Management

Exercise 5-1 Patient Care and Management

DIRECTIONS: Use each answer only once.

A. Purulent
B. Antecubital
C. Nocturia
D. Infiltrated
E. Nasogastric (NG)
F. Lateral
G. Rheumatoid arthritis
H. Logrolling
I. Neurogenic
J. Urinary tract infection (UTI)
K. Reflux
L. Kitoacidosis
M. Epinephrine
N. Bolus
O. Pelvis
P. Contact isolation
Q. Carcinoma
R. Incubation period
S. Septic
T. Sarcoma
U. Acetaminophen
V. Surgical asepsis
W. Aspiration
X. Exudate
Y. Strict Isolation

_____ 1. Utilized for diseases spread by close or direct contact
_____ 2. First stage of an infection
_____ 3. Cancer derived from epithelial tissue
_____ 4. Shock caused by severe systemic infection
_____ 5. Most common nosacomial infection
_____ 6. Bronchodilator and vasoconstrictive drug
_____ 7. Center of gravity when person is standing
_____ 8 Tube inserted into the stomach for decompression
_____ 9. Types of fluid with a high content of cellular material
_____ 10. Swelling at site of needle insertion
_____ 11. Complete removal of all microorganisms from an object
_____ 12. Cancer derived from connective tissue
_____ 13. Most required for patients with airborne or contact route diseases
_____ 14. Common vein for intravenous administration
_____ 15. Drawing in: inhaling or drawing out by suction
_____ 16. Inflammatory overgrowth of the synovial tissue
_____ 17. Drug given to a patient's preexisting intravenous
_____ 18. Orally taken drug that treats pain without anti-inflammatory effects
_____ 19. Diabetic patients with lack of insulin have an attack of
_____ 20. Used to move patients with spine injuries
_____ 21. Shock occurring with spinal cord injury
_____ 22. Producing or containing pus
_____ 23. Excessive urination at night
_____ 24. Backward flow that is usually unnatural
_____ 25. Position to place patient who begins to vomit

Answer Key	Notes
1. P	
2. R	
3. Q	
4. S	
5. J	
6. M	
7. O	
8. E	
9. X	
10. D	
11. V	
12. T	
13. Y	
14. B	
15. W	
16. G	
17. N	
18. U	
19. L	
20. H	
21. I	
22. A	
23. C	
24. K	
25. F	

Exercise **5-2** # Medicolegal Terms

DIRECTIONS: Use each answer only once.

A. Felony
B. Defamation
C. Tort
D. Common law
E. Juris prudence
F. Libel
G. Civil law
H. Malfeasance
I. Slander
J. Burden of proof
K. Res judicata
L. Feasance
M. Rule of discovery
N. Noncomposmentis
O. Contributory negligence
P. Medical audit
Q. Misfeasance
R. Invasion of privacy
S. Plaintiff
T. Criminal law
U. Nonfeasance
V. Res ipsa loquitur
W. Statute of limitations
X. Defendant
Y. Judicial

_____ 1. Person who brings an action
_____ 2. Private or civil wrong or injury
_____ 3. Philosophy of law
_____ 4. Defamatory words that are printed
_____ 5. Offense of injuring another's reputation
_____ 6. Relating to or connected with the administration of justice
_____ 7. Law that deals with conduct offensive to society
_____ 8. Doing an act that is wrongful and unlawful
_____ 9. Legal limit on the time one has to file suit
_____ 10. Judge-made law from common court decision
_____ 11. Encroachment on the right of privacy
_____ 12. Oral defamation: speaking falsely about another
_____ 13. Improper performance of some act you can by law do
_____ 14. Enforcement of civil rights as distinguished from criminal law
_____ 15. Person defending or denying
_____ 16. Affirmatively proving a fact
_____ 17. Crime of a grave or atrocious nature
_____ 18. Omission of an act that a person ought to do
_____ 19. Matter judged or judicially acted upon
_____ 20. Omission of performing ordinary care
_____ 21. The thing speaks for itself
_____ 22. Not sound of mind; insane
_____ 23. Performance of an act
_____ 24. Statute of limitations that does not begin to run until patient knows
_____ 25. Study of patient's records to assess care

Answer Key	Notes
1. S	
2. C	
3. E	
4. F	
5. B	
6. Y	
7. T	
8. H	
9. W	
10. D	
11. R	
12. I	
13. Q	
14. G	
15. X	
16. J	
17. A	
18. U	
19. K	
20. O	
21. V	
22. N	
23. L	
24. M	
25. P	

Exercise 5-3 Medical Abbreviations

DIRECTIONS: Use each answer only once.

A. QAM
B. METS
C. MM
D. NA
E. Grav 1,2,3
F. BX
G. Per os (PO)
H. HX
I. PO 2
J. CHR
K. QHS
L. CXR
M. Q
N. ASA
O. MMHG
P. H/O
Q. DX
R. OD
S. C.F.
T. OZ
U. K
V. G
W. Rx
X. MCG
Y. TX

_____ 1. Diagnosis
_____ 2. Right eye
_____ 3. By mouth
_____ 4. Aspirin
_____ 5. Every morning
_____ 6. History of
_____ 7. Treatment
_____ 8. Chest x-ray
_____ 9. Microgram
_____ 10. Pregnant (gravida)
_____ 11. Treatment, prescription
_____ 12. Biopsy
_____ 13. Each bedtime
_____ 14. 1/1000 m
_____ 15. Sodium,
_____ 16. Potassium
_____ 17. Compare
_____ 18. Mestastases
_____ 19. History
_____ 20. Oxygen pressure
_____ 21. Long term; chronic
_____ 22. Ounce
_____ 23. First, second, third pregnancy
_____ 24. Each, every
_____ 25. Millimeters of mercury

Answer Key	Notes
1. Q	
2. R	
3. G	
4. N	
5. A	
6. P	
7. Y	
8. L	
9. X	
10. V	
11. W	
12. F	
13. K	
14. C	
15. D	
16. U	
17. S	
18. B	
19. H	
20. I	
21. J	
22. T	
23. E	
24. M	
25. O	

Exercise 5-4 Abbreviations

DIRECTIONS: Use each answer only once.

A. STAT
B. FB
C. Port
D. SID
E. FSS
F. FX
G. IM
H. BP
I. N.P.O.
J. c̄
K. DOA
L. O_2
M. URC
N. RT (R)
O. T.I.D.
P. IBA
Q. PRN
R. s̄
S. Q.I.D.
T. H.U.
U. cm
V. PT
W. B.I.D.
X. OTO
Y. P.I.

_____ 1. Patient will be admitted to floor
_____ 2. Reading of systolic and diasystolic pressure
_____ 3. Individual being treated
_____ 4. Relating to ear
_____ 5. Three times a day
_____ 6. Term for something not normally seen on film
_____ 7. As needed
_____ 8. Measurement used in radiography
_____ 9. Without
_____ 10. Four times a day
_____ 11. ARRT certification in radiography
_____ 12. Measure of heat by multiplying mAs × kVp
_____ 13. Immediately
_____ 14. Illness patient is experiencing
_____ 15. Twice a day
_____ 16. AMA accreditation agency
_____ 17. Fasting for examination
_____ 18. With
_____ 19. Term for "fracture"
_____ 20. Referring to target
_____ 21. Same as TFD or FFD
_____ 22. Patient arrives dead
_____ 23. Oxygen
_____ 24. Bedside radiograph
_____ 25. Injection given in muscle

Answer Key	Notes
1. P	
2. H	
3. V	
4. X	
5. O	
6. B	
7. Q	
8. U	
9. R	
10. S	
11. N	
12. T	
13. A	
14. Y	
15. W	
16. M	
17. I	
18. J	
19. F	
20. E	
21. D	
22. K	
23. L	
24. C	
25. G	

Exercise 5-5 Medical Ethics and Law

DIRECTIONS: Use each answer only once.

A. Informed consent
B. Ethics
C. Revocation
D. Endorser
E. Malpractice
F. Annotate
G. Power of attorney
H. Assault
I. Perjured testimony
J. Dilemma
K. Pejorative
L. Bias
M. Third party payer
N. Discretion
O. Prerogative
P. Protocols
Q. Battery
R. Statutory body
S. Liability
T. Substantiated
U. Prudent
V. Litigation
W. Quackery
X. Therapeutic
Y. Treatise

_____ 1. Inclination or temperament based on personal judgment
_____ 2. Telling what is false when sworn to tell the truth
_____ 3. Established as true by competent evidence
_____ 4. Intentional, unlawful attempt to injure
_____ 5. Contest in court for the purpose of enforcing right
_____ 6. Consent involving an understanding of risks and procedure
_____ 7. Systematic exposition or argument in writing
_____ 8. Willful and unlawful use of force or violence
_____ 9. Legal statement authorizing another person to act as an agent
_____ 10. Person who signs his or her name to the back of a check
_____ 11. Acceptable, professional mode of behavior
_____ 12. Act of annulling by recalling or taking back
_____ 13. Quality of being tactful or prudent
_____ 14. Exclusive and unquestionable right belonging to a person
_____ 15. To furnish with explanatory notes
_____ 16. Pretense of medical skill
_____ 17. Professional misconduct, improper discharge of duties
_____ 18. Situation involving choice between equally unsatisfactory alternatives
_____ 19. Capable of directing oneself wisely and judiciously
_____ 20. Having negative connotations, a depreciatory word
_____ 21. Part of the legislative branch of a government
_____ 22. State or quality of being responsible for
_____ 23. Pertaining to the art of healing, curative
_____ 24. Rules of performance
_____ 25. Someone other than patient responsible for the bill

Answer Key	Notes
1. L	
2. I	
3. T	
4. H	
5. V	
6. A	
7. Y	
8. Q	
9. G	
10. D	
11. B	
12. C	
13. N	
14. O	
15. F	
16. W	
17. E	
18. J	
19. U	
20. K	
21. R	
22. S	
23. X	
24. P	
25. M	

Exercise 5-6 Law and Ethics

DIRECTIONS: Use each answer only once.

A. Confidentiality
B. Breach
C. Reasonable cause
D. Adjudicated
E. Deposition
F. Due care
G. Cognitive
H. Evidence
I. Civil
J. Grossly negligent
K. Assets
L. Fraud
M. Conspiring
N. Implied
O. Credibility
P. Burden of proof
Q. Restraint
R. Principal
S. Vicariously liable
T. Capacity
U. Subpoena
V. Malice
W. Undue influence
X. Wanton
Y. Fiduciary

_____ 1. Legally obligated in place of someone else
_____ 2. Type of proof presented by a witness in court
_____ 3. Personal belongings and property owned by a person
_____ 4. Improper persuasion to make someone act differently
_____ 5. Pertaining to crimes against a person or persons
_____ 6. Acceptable degree of care under certain circumstances
_____ 7. Necessity of giving convincing legal proof of facts
_____ 8. Prior statement by a witness in court under oath
_____ 9. Not indicated by direct words but evident from conduct
_____ 10. Heard and settled by a judicial process
_____ 11. Employer, or source of authority of the agent
_____ 12. State of being treated as a private matter
_____ 13. Unlawful violation of an obligation or contract
_____ 14. Branch of government that interprets and applies the law
_____ 15. Relating to knowledge
_____ 16. Command to appear at a place to testify
_____ 17. Secretly planning to perform an illegal act
_____ 18. Restriction of liberty
_____ 19. Qualification to understand the results of an action
_____ 20. Failing intentionally to perform a necessary duty
_____ 21. To have adequate regard for someone's rights
_____ 22. Quality in a witness that makes the person believable
_____ 23. Unjust intention to commit an illegal act or injury
_____ 24. Deliberate deception
_____ 25. Done with reckless disregard of another's rights

Answer Key	Notes
1. S	
2. H	
3. K	
4. W	
5. I	
6. C	
7. P	
8. E	
9. N	
10. D	
11. R	
12. A	
13. B	
14. Y	
15. G	
16. U	
17. M	
18. Q	
19. T	
20. J	
21. F	
22. O	
23. V	
24. L	
25. X	

Exercise 5-7 Nursing Information

DIRECTIONS: Use each answer only once.

A. Cytotoxic
B. Heparin
C. Antiinflammatories
D. Diuretic
E. Cathartics
F. Achalasia
G. Hemostatics
H. Antidepressants
I. Expectorants
J. Digitalis
K. Antiarrhythmics
L. Lymphosarcoma
M. Antiflatulents
N. Antipruritics
O. Hypertension
P. Antiseptics
Q. Intussusception
R. Anticholinergics
S. Agenesis
T. Tranquilizers
U. Antitussives
V. Astringents
W. Hernia
X. Dulcolax
Y. Cardio Tonics

_____ 1. Mood elevators
_____ 2. Stop and control bleeding or hemorrhage
_____ 3.. Bowel cleanser
_____ 4. Failure of esophagus to relax
_____ 5. Relieve itching
_____ 6. Prevents blood clotting
_____ 7. Invagination of a portion of intestine
_____ 8. Cause the bowel to evacuate its contents
_____ 9. Blood pressure elevation: 140+ systole, 95+ diastolic
_____ 10. Defective development or absence of an organ
_____ 11. Cough suppressant in allergies
_____ 12. Increases urine output
_____ 13. Used for skin cleaning
_____ 14. Protrusion of a loop of an organ through an opening
_____ 15. Primary or metastic tumor
_____ 16. Increases strength of myocardiac contraction
_____ 17. Stops bleeding from minor cuts
_____ 18. Common cardiac stimulant
_____ 19. Acts to regulate heart beat
_____ 20. Act as central nervous system depressant
_____ 21. Relief of gastric or intestinal gas
_____ 22. Drugs used to destroy particular cells in cancer treatment
_____ 23. Treats bronchitis and other respiratory conditions
_____ 24. Reduces muscle spasms
_____ 25. Act to diminish inflammation

Answer Key	Notes
1. H	
2. G	
3. X	
4. F	
5. N	
6. B	
7. Q	
8. E	
9. O	
10. S	
11. U	
12. D	
13. P	
14. W	
15. L	
16. Y	
17. V	
18. J	
19. K	
20. T	
21. M	
22. A	
23. I	
24. R	
25. C	

Exercise 5-8 Nursing Information

DIRECTIONS: Use each answer only once.

A. Hemiplegic
B. Simethicone
C. Anaphylaxis
D. Hemoptysis
E. Cyanosis
F. Hypovolemic
G. Adrenalin
H. Analgesic
I. Glucagon
J. Insulin
K. Emetics
L. Epistaxis
M. Sedative
N. 50% glucose
O. Antiemetic
P. Anorexia
Q. Antibiotic
R. Vasoconstrictor
S. Nitroglycerin
T. Anticoagulent
U. Vasodilator
V. Hypnotic
W. Paraplegic
X. Percodan
Y. Vertigo

_____ 1. Dizziness
_____ 2. Paralysis to lower half of body
_____ 3. Loss of appetite
_____ 4. Used for diabetic shock
_____ 5. Prevents clotting of blood
_____ 6. Nosebleed
_____ 7. Stops vomiting
_____ 8. Used for diabetic coma
_____ 9. Helps to relax
_____ 10. Paralysis to one side of body
_____ 11. Narrows blood vessels
_____ 12. Drug used to raise blood pressure
_____ 13. Used for pain control as an opiate
_____ 14. Produces sleep
_____ 15. Pancreatic extract
_____ 16. Used for cardiac pain
_____ 17. Enlarges blood vessels
_____ 18. Drug to relieve pain
_____ 19. Spitting up of blood
_____ 20. Blueness due to lack of O_2
_____ 21. Shock associated with massive blood loss
_____ 22. Used to relieve gastric acidity
_____ 23. Induces vomiting
_____ 24. Allergy to CM injection
_____ 25. Fights infection

Answer Key	Notes
1. Y	
2. W	
3. P	
4. N	
5. T	
6. L	
7. O	
8. S	
9. M	
10. A	
11. R	
12. G	
13. X	
14. V	
15. I	
16. S	
17. U	
18. H	
19. D	
20. E	
21. F	
22. B	
23. K	
24. C	
25. Q	

Exercise 5-9 Vital Signs

DIRECTIONS: Use each answer only once.

A. 10 to 20
B. 99 degrees
C. Cardinal signs
D. Palliative
E. 97.6 degrees
F. Apical
G. Popliteal
H. 120 beats/min
I. 99.6 degrees
J. Radial
K. Pulse
L. Systolic
M. 98.6 degrees
N. 30 to 60
O. 60 to 90 beats/min
P. 140+ over 90
Q. 97.8 degrees
R. Sphygmomanometer
S. Diastolic
T. Fever
U. 100 to 140 mmHg
V. Lentigines
W. 60 to 80 mmHg
X. 90 to 100 beats/min
Y. 90 mmHg (systolic)

_____ 1. Most accurate pulse location for infants and children
_____ 2. Throb felt on an artery
_____ 3. Average adult breaths/minute
_____ 4. Pulse found on posterior surface of knee
_____ 5 Normal rectal temperature
_____ 6. Normal systolic pressure
_____ 7. Disturbance in heat-regulating centers
_____ 8. Average body temperature from 3 months to 3 years
_____ 9. Average infant respirations/min
_____ 10. Normal axillary temperature
_____ 11. Round, flat brown pigmented spot on the skin
_____ 12. Patient considered to be hypotensive
_____ 13. Normal body temperature 5 to 13 years of age
_____ 14. Normal diastolic pressure
_____ 15. Decreases pain
_____ 16. Highest point reached during contraction of left ventricle
_____ 17. Normal oral temperature
_____ 18. Average pulse rate for an infant
_____ 19. Most accessible and convenient pulse location
_____ 20. Lowest point of pressure during ventricle relaxation
_____ 21. Another name for vital signs
_____ 22. Patient considered hypertensive
_____ 23. Average adult (resting) pulse rate
_____ 24. Blood pressure instrument
_____ 25. Average 4 to 10-year-old pulse rate

Answer Key	Notes
1. F	
2. K	
3. A	
4. G	
5. I	
6. U	
7. T	
8. B	
9. N	
10. E	
11. V	
12. Y	
13. Q	
14. W	
15. D	
16. L	
17. M	
18. H	
19. J	
20. S	
21. C	
22. P	
23. O	
24. R	
25. X	

Exercise 5-10 Contrast Media Administration

DIRECTIONS: Answers may be used more than once.

A. Invasive injection
B. Ingestion
C. Induction
D. Catheter injection (noninvasive)

_____ 1. Esophagram
_____ 2. Endoscopy
_____ 3. Oral cholecystography
_____ 4. T-tube cholangiography
_____ 5. Retrograde pyelogram
_____ 6. Sialography
_____ 7. Bronchography
_____ 8. GI series
_____ 9. Percutaneous transhepatic cholangiography
_____ 10. Barium enema
_____ 11. Cardiac series
_____ 12. IVP
_____ 13. Arch aortography
_____ 14. Small bowel series
_____ 15. Pneumoencephalography
_____ 16. Veinography
_____ 17. Cystogram
_____ 18. Herniography
_____ 19. Surgical cholangiography
_____ 20. Arthrography
_____ 21. Myelography
_____ 22. Pneumoventriculography
_____ 23. Hysterosalpingogram
_____ 24. Thoracic aortography
_____ 25. Angiography

Answer Key	Notes
1. B	
2. D	
3. B	
4. D	
5. D	
6. C	
7. D	
8. B	
9. A	
10. C	
11. B	
12. A	
13. A	
14. B	
15. A	
16. A	
17. D	
18. A	
19. A	
20. A	
21. A	
22. A	
23. D	
24. A	
25. A	

Exercise 5-11 Contrast Media and Medications

DIRECTIONS: Answers may be used more than once. Items can require more than one answer (CM=contrast media).

A. Ethiodol
B. Telepaque
C. Procaine
D. Paque Panto (iohexol)
E. Dionosil
F. Hypaque
G. Salpix
H. $BaSO_4$
I. Esophatrast
J. Gastrografin
K. Ethiodized oil
L. Benadryl
M. Aminophyline
N. Atrophine
O. Neocholex
P. Betadine
Q. Bisadodyl
R. Heparin
S. Amipaque
T. Ammonia spirits
U. Orografin
V. Dextrose in water
W. Nitroglycerin
X. Metrizamide
Y. Saline

_____ 1. Drug taken for chest pain
_____ 2. Used for fainting
_____ 3. Hysterosalpingography (cm)
_____ 4. Myelogram (cm)
_____ 5. Stomach with perforation (cm)
_____ 6. Used in gastric disease as an antispasmotic and antisecretion
_____ 7. Contrast agent used in lymphography
_____ 8. Intestinal tract contrast media
_____ 9. Local anesthetic
_____ 10. Esophagus contrast agent
_____ 11. Kidneys and ureters (cm)
_____ 12. Salpingography (cm)
_____ 13. Administered for anaphylaxis
_____ 14. Oral cholecystogram (cm)
_____ 15. Bronchography (cm)
_____ 16. Used to prevent blood clotting
_____ 17. Pneumo arthrograms (cm)
_____ 18. Salt water used in intravenous injections
_____ 19. Releases bronchial smooth muscle management
_____ 20. Cholecystagogue use with gallbladder
_____ 21. Spinal column (cm)
_____ 22. Cathartic preparation
_____ 23. Antiseptic for skin preparation
_____ 24 Intravenous nutrient
_____ 25. Utilized in hypoglycemia

Answer Key	Notes
1. W	
2. T	
3. G/A	
4. D/X	
5. J	
6. N	
7. K	
8. H	
9. C	
10. I	
11. F	
12. A/G	
13. L	
14. U/B	
15. E	
16. R	
17. K	
18. Y	
19. M	
20. O	
21. D/X	
22. Q	
23. P	
24. V	
25. M	

Exercise 5-12 Contrast Media Reactions and Procedures

A. Mild
B. Moderate
C. Severe
D. Invasive
E. Noninvasive

DIRECTIONS: In items 1 to 15, match the appropriate level of reaction. Use choices A, B, or C. Answers may be used more than once.

_____ 1. Tachycardia
_____ 2. Itching
_____ 3. Convulsions
_____ 4. Sneezing
_____ 5. Cyanosis
_____ 6. Nausea and Vomiting
_____ 7. Excessive vomiting
_____ 8. Dyspnea
_____ 9. Urticaria (mild)
_____ 10. Laryngeal edema
_____ 11. Vasovagal response
_____ 12. Very low blood pressure
_____ 13. Burning or numbness at injection site
_____ 14. Loss of consciousness
_____ 15. Giant hives

DIRECTIONS: In items 16 to 24, identify as invasive or noninvasive procedures. Use choices D and E. Answers may be used more than once.

_____ 16. Arthrography
_____ 17. Angiography
_____ 18. Cholecystography
_____ 19. Esophagram
_____ 20. Gastrointestinal series
_____ 21. Urography
_____ 22. Cholangiography
_____ 23. Myelography
_____ 24. Barium enema

Answer Key	Notes
1. B	
2. A	
3. C	
4. A	
5. C	
6. A	
7. B	
8. C	
9. A	
10. C	
11. A	
12. C	
13. A	
14. C	
15. B	
16. D	
17. D	
18. E	
19. E	
20. E	
21. D	
22. D	
23. D	
24. E	

Exercise 5-13 Infection Control

DIRECTIONS: Use each answer only once.

A. Antibody
B. Cytotoxic
C. Droplet contact
D. Pathogenic
E. Contaminate
F. Nosocomial infections
G. Vehicle contact
H. Indirect contact
I. Incubation
J. Protozoa
K. Viruses
L. Antigen
M. Bacteria
N. Active
O. Hands
P. Immunosuppressive
Q. Interferon
R. Direct contact
S. Fungi
T. Airborne contact
U. Prodromal
V. Fomites
W. Remission
X. Host
Y. Convalescence

_____ 1. Capable of producing a disease
_____ 2. Microorganism unresponsive to antibacterial drugs
_____ 3. Complex one-celled microorganisms
_____ 4. Period when symptoms of disease are not apparent
_____ 5. Introduction of microorganisms into a clean area
_____ 6. Foreign protein
_____ 7. Minute organisms without a typical nucleus
_____ 8. Most common means of spreading infection
_____ 9. Second phase of an infection
_____ 10. Inhaling air contaminated with infectious microbe
_____ 11. Third phase of an infection
_____ 12. Purpose of hospital infection control is to prevent
_____ 13. Objects contaminated by an infected person
_____ 14. Drugs used to destroy/prevent cell multiplication
_____ 15. Ingesting contaminated water, food, drugs, or blood
_____ 16. Protein globulin produced by specific cells
_____ 17. Contact with secretions by sneezing–coughing–talk
_____ 18. Period of recovery at the end of a disease
_____ 19. Person susceptible to infection
_____ 20. Touching contaminated objects with microbe
_____ 21. First stage in the course of an infection
_____ 22. Reproducing yeasts and molds by spore formation
_____ 23. Drugs that interfere with normal immune response
_____ 24. Touching contaminated materials with hands
_____ 25. Restores body's immune systems following foreign agent attack

Answer Key

Notes

1. D
2. K
3. J
4. W
5. E
6. L
7. M
8. O
9. U
10. T
11. N
12. F
13. V
14. B
15. G
16. A
17. C
18. Y
19. X
20. R
21. I
22. S
23. P
24. H
25. Q

Exercise 5-14 Medical Emergencies

DIRECTIONS: Use each answer only once.

A. Hyperosmolar coma
B. 12 per minute
C. Fainting
D. Circulation
E. Xiphoid process
F. Shock
G. Carotid
H. 80 to 100
I. CVA
J. Open airway
K. Comatose
L. Diabetic coma
M. 7 sec
N. 15
O. T.I.A.
P. Breathing
Q. Lethargy
R. 1½ to 2 in.
S. Epilepsy
T. Hyperextension
U. Urticaria
V. Diabetic ketoacidosis
W. Pallor
X. Hypoglycemia
Y. Diaphoresis

_____ 1. Occlusion or rupture of cerebral arteries
_____ 2. Third step required during CPR
_____ 3. Mild type of stroke
_____ 4. First action for respiratory or cardiac arrest
_____ 5. Absence or lack of skin color
_____ 6. Chest compressions for every two inflations
_____ 7. Most common convulsive seizure
_____ 8. Breathing rates administered to an adult
_____ 9. Complication of diabetes melitus
_____ 10. Occurs when insufficient insulin is present in body
_____ 11. Pulse checked during CPR
_____ 12. Disturbance of blood flow to vital organs
_____ 13. Hands for chest massage are above
_____ 14. Caused by insufficient blood to the brain
_____ 15. Second action: for respiratory or cardiac arrest
_____ 16. Profuse sweating
_____ 17. Patient administered 20 to 50 mL of 50% glucose
_____ 18. Position of head during mouth-to-mouth breathing
_____ 19. Abnormal deep stupor
_____ 20. External chest compression per minute for an adult
_____ 21. Compressions of chest should not be interrupted for
_____ 22. Occurs in diabetics with excess amounts of insulin in blood
_____ 23 Compression required for an adult chest
_____ 24. Giant hives resulting from allergic reaction
_____ 25. Condition of indifference or suppression of emotions

Answer Key	Notes
1. I	
2. D	
3. O	
4. J	
5. W	
6. N	
7. S	
8. B	
9. A	
10. V	
11. G	
12. F	
13. E	
14. C	
15. P	
16. Y	
17. L	
18. T	
19. K	
20. H	
21. M	
22. X	
23. R	
24. U	
25. Q	

References

Anderson, K. N., and Anderson, L. E. (1990). *Mosby's Pocket Dictionary of Medicine, Nursing, and Allied Health*. St. Louis, MO.: Mosby-Year Book, Inc.

Armstrong, P. and Wastie, M. (1992). *Diagnostic Imaging*, 3rd Edition. Cambridge, Mass.: Blackwell Scientific Publications, Inc.

Ballinger, P. W. (1991). *Merrill's Atlas of Radiologic Positions and Radiographic Procedures*, 7th Edition. St. Louis, MO.: Mosby-Year Book, Inc.

Ballinger, P. W. (1992). *Pocket Guide to Radiography*, 2nd Edition. St. Louis, MO.: Mosby-Year Book, Inc.

Bontrager, K., and Anthony, B. T. (1993). *Textbook of Radiography Positioning and Related Anatomy*, 3rd Edition. St. Louis, MO.: Mosby-Year Book, Inc.

Burke, S. (1992). *Human Anatomy and Physiology in Health and Disease*, 3rd Edition. Albany, N.Y.: Delmar Publishers, Inc.

Bushong, S. (1993). *Radiologic Science for Technologists*, 5th Edition. St. Louis, MO.: Mosby-Year Book, Inc.

Campeau, F. and Phelps, M. (1993). *Limited Radiography*. Albany, N.Y.: Delmar Publishers, Inc.

Carlton, R. and Adler, A. (1992). *Principles of Radiographing Imaging*. Albany, N.Y.: Delmar Publishers, Inc.

Cullinan, A. (1992). *Optimizing Radiographic Positioning*. Philadelphia: J. B. Lippincott Company.

Cullinan, A. (1987). *Producing Quality Radiographs*. Philadelphia: J. B. Lippincott Company.

Donohue, D. P. (1984). *An Analysis of Radiographic Quality*. Rockville, MD.: Aspen Systems, Inc.

Drafke, M. (1990). *Trauma and Mobile Radiography*. Philadelphia: F. A. Davis Company.

Ehrlich, A. (1988). *Medical Terminology for Health Professions*. Albany, N.Y.: Delmar Publishers, Inc.

Ehrlich, R., and McCloskey, E. (1989). *Patient Care in Radiography*, 3rd Edition. St. Louis, MO.: Mosby-Year Book, Inc.

Eisenberg, R. L., Dennis, C., and May, C. (1989). *Radiographic Positioning*. Boston: Little, Brown & Co., Inc.

Fiesta, J. (1988). *The Law and Liability: A Guide for Nurses*, 2nd Edition. New York: John Wiley & Sons, Inc.

Gurley, L. T., and Callaway, W. J. (1992). *Introduction to Radiologic Technology*, 3rd Edition. St. Louis, MO.: Mosby-Year Book, Inc.

Laudicina, P. (1989). *Applied Pathology for Radiographers.* Philadelphia: W. B. Saunders Company.

Loebel, S. (1991). *The Nurse's Drug Handbook*, 6th Edition. Albany, N.Y.: Delmar Publishers, Inc.

Mace, J. D., and Kowalczyk, N. (1988). *Radiographic Pathology for Technologists.* St. Louis, MO.: Mosby-Year Book, Inc.

Martini, F. (1992). *Fundamentals of Anatomy and Physiology*, 2nd Edition. Englewood Cliffs, N.J.: Prentice Hall.

Miller, B. F., and Keane, C. B. (1992). *Encyclopedia and Dictionary of Medicine, Nursing, and Allied Health,* 5th Edition. Philadelphia: W. B. Saunders Company.

Rambo, B. J., and Wood, L. A. (1982). *Nursing Skills for Clinical Practice,* 3rd Edition. Philadelphia: W. B. Saunders Company.

Snopeck, A. (1992). *Fundamentals of Special Radiographic Procedures,* 3rd Edition. Philadelphia: W. B. Saunders Company.

Statkiewicz, M., and Ritenour, E. (1983). *Radiation Protection for Student Radiographers.* Denver, CO.: Multi Media Publishing.

Sweeney, R. (1983). *Radiographic Artifacts: Their Cause and Control.* Philadelphia: J. B. Lippincott Company.

Thompson, T. T. (1979). *Cahoon's Formulating X-Ray Techniques,* 9th Edition. Durham, N.C.: Duke University Press.

Torres, L. (1989). *Basic Medical Techniques and Patient Care for Radiologic Technologists,* 3rd Edition. Philadelphia: J. B. Lippincott Company.

Tortora, G, and Anagnostakos, N. (1990). *Principles of Anatomy and Physiology,* 6th Edition. New York: Harper Collins Publishers.

Tortorici, M. (1992). *Concepts in Medical Radiographic Imaging.* Philadelphia: W. B. Saunders Company.

Wicke, L. (1987). *Atlas of Radiologic Anatomy,* 4th Edition. Baltimore: Urban & Schwarzenberg, Inc.